WEIGHT CONTROL *That Works*

10 Daily Habits to Lose Weight, Keep it Off & Love Your Body

Christie Jordan

A Hopeful Woman Book

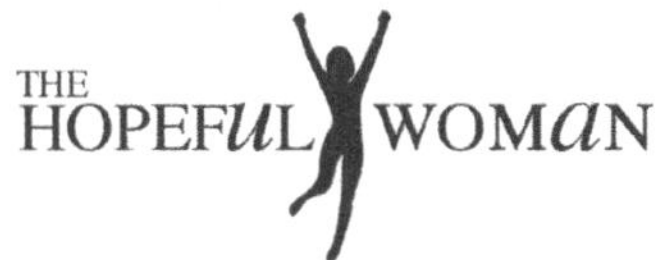

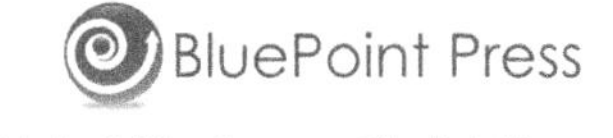

Orinda, California   www.BluePointPress.com

WEIGHT CONTROL THAT WORKS:
10 DAILY HABITS TO LOSE WEIGHT,
KEEP IT OFF & LOVE YOUR BODY

2nd Edition Softcover ISBN: 978-0-9890106-2-7
Previously published under ISBN: 978-0-9890106-0-3
eBook ISBN: 978-0-9890106-1-0
1. Reducing diets. 2. Food habits. 3. Nutrition. 4. Weight loss. 5. Title.
Library of Congress Cataloging-in-Publication Data is available upon request.

Interior Design by Lisa DeSpain, ebookconverting.com

PRAISE FOR WEIGHT CONTROL THAT WORKS

"No one understands how to keep weight off better than someone who has struggled with dieting for years, then lost 85 pounds and sustained it by changing her lifestyle.

"As a health care provider, I really appreciate Christie's focus on an up-to-date scientific understanding of the topic and her patient, practical advice about how changes in nutrition and lifestyle can make a big difference in overall health.

"This book is both optimistic and realistic! Thank you, Christie, for sharing what you've learned!"

Ann C. Tipton, M.D.

"This book is your tool box for making lasting change in your life and in your weight control. As a Clinical Nutritionist, assisting clients through lifestyle changes has been the cornerstone and most successful approach to lasting results. You now have the tools in the palm of your hand to make those changes. It's written in an understandable, complete and friendly way. I think you will feel empowered by this book."

Roxanne Curley, Clinical Nutritionist

"Yo-yo diets made me desperate for a better way. Here it is!"

Lianna Moore, Creative Director

"You won't find a more comprehensive book about how to control your weight. From hormones to the Glycemic Index to fidgeting for extra exercise, Christie Jordan has done a wonderful job of organizing complex, research-based information for you to read and understand."

Audra Willeke, PhD, University Professor

"Finally, a book that clearly gives the information that I have tried to convey to many of my therapy clients for a long time. Christie has written an easy to read and interesting book. She has shown us a clear way to stay healthy and fit. Don't miss reading this fun and informative book."

Laurel Rose, MFTT, Licensed Marriage and Family Therapist

"A mix of personal stories and scientific research that offers creative tips and humor you won't find in other weight control books or programs.

"Readers will benefit from Christie's unshakeable faith that she could lose 85 pounds and keep it off for 18 years. Her creative tips and humor will help you live long enough to play with your grandchildren!

"My father used to say, 'If you get one new idea from a book, it was worth reading.' This book passes the test. Christie offers many creative ideas for reaching and maintaining a healthy weight. An important contribution to an increasingly obese America."

Shelley O'Connor, Attorney

"If you want to optimize your ability to lose weight and keep it off, this book is a must-read."

Shimyun Cotter, MA, High School Teacher

"In a crowded field of books about losing weight, this book really stands out as different because the focus is making weight loss permanent. The chapters are well organized and all recommendations are backed up with solid information about nutrition and plenty of practical, hands-on suggestions you can apply to your daily life.

"This is not an ordinary diet book! Learning the weight control lifestyle is your roadmap to healthy living and success in keeping those pounds off."

Winfried Wilcke, PhD, Scientist

"Having seen a proof copy of *Weight Control That Works*, at first I thought that another diet book is just overkill. That market is saturated. However, this book takes a new and refreshing look at the obesity epidemic and focuses on keeping weight off. As I checked the *10 Daily Habits*, I said to myself, 'I've done that. And then, oh well, I _could_ do that.'

"I am especially impressed with the book design and layout. Lists really help me. The textbook style makes it easy to focus on the areas I need the most. The 'Learn More' bits feed my curiosity and interest in deeper explanations. The book is also easy to read, concise, and appeals to my sense of humor."

Geraldine Tiziani, MS, LMS, Library Media Specialist

For my sons, Christopher & Jonathan

*Who are my inspiration to take good care
of myself so I'll be here for their future*

And For Hopeful Women Everywhere

*Who have the courage and determination
to reinvent their lives.
Believe in your own strength!*

CONTENTS

PART ONE:
START BY LEARNING WHY YOU ARE UNIQUE

Only you have your unique combination of genetic inheritance, metabolism, childhood training and current lifestyle.

PART TWO:
10 DAILY HABITS FOR
WEIGHT CONTROL THAT WORKS

Willpower and appetite are affected by lack of sleep.

Getting enough sleep is a must for weight control.

Eat a breakfast with protein and whole grains to jump-start your metabolism.

What to stock in your kitchen.

PART FOUR:
4 BONUS HABITS

If the food has a label, never put it in your mouth until you read it.

Ignore sales slogans.

Become more aware of how you're eating and drinking. Loose twice as much weight! Help transition from unhealthy eating habits to a lifestyle that supports weight control.

Repeating meals saves you time and money.

Recipes for breakfast and lunch.

You deserve praise for working to improve your health. If you stumble, recommit to your longterm goal of weight control and move forward.

Never give up!

PART FIVE:
RESOURCES FOR LEARNING MORE

INTRODUCTION

This book is about how I lost 85 pounds and kept them off.

Most people who diet for weight loss gain the weight right back, but if you change your lifestyle with new habits, permanent weight control is possible. I've done it, and you can do it, too!

Have you struggled to control your weight, gaining and losing then gaining again? Do you dread getting on a scale or finding an outfit for a special party? And what about that doctor visit? What if you were told that you now have a true health issue—not just concerns about how you look—because of your extra weight?

Well, I've been there.

I was seriously overweight until I was fifty years old. More than one doctor told me that I was morbidly obese and should do something about it. So, for decades I followed fad diets, lost weight then embarrassed myself when the pounds came quickly back. I finally lost 85 pounds permanently by putting together a collection of habits, helpful tricks and changes in attitude that made it possible to master weight control in a way that is healthy for my body and comfortable for my lifestyle.

It was a long process for me, with lots of trial and error until I figured out what worked to keep me healthy and my weight under control. How I wish there had been a book like this to guide me! But here it is, and I hope this book will give you the help you need.

You can break the cycle of losing and gaining weight and finally stop dieting.

You can learn to be comfortable and relaxed with your body and your relationship with food.

How do I know that my weight loss is permanent?

After a lifetime of yo-yo dieting, how can I be so sure that the 85 pounds I lost won't come back like so many times before? How can I feel confident that not even 20 or 30 pounds will slip back on? It's because my weight has been stable for 18 years. I went from a size 24 to a size 8 and have stayed there. Control is no longer a constant challenge. Sure, like anyone, I've gained five pounds or more on vacation, but once that time is over, I carefully follow the 10 Daily Habits and watch my calorie intake until I'm back at my goal weight.

I even lived through menopause without gaining weight, hot flashes and all! I live comfortably with my eating and exercise habits. Feeling relaxed and confident about what I do keeps me in good shape and feeling happy about how I look and feel.

I would love to share what I've learned with you.

This is not a diet book

That's right. You will lose weight by following the 10 Daily Habits for Weight Control, but this is not a book about how to lose weight fast. It's a book about lifestyle habits, which will gradually drop extra pounds and keep them off comfortably. If you follow this collection of practical tips, techniques and—most importantly—habits you will learn to overcome cravings, break the patterns of unhealthy eating and stay motivated.

This book is filled with real-life techniques you can use to finally master controlling your weight for the rest of your life. There is much to learn in these pages.

Thirty-five years of experience is here for you

Between being a chubby teenager and an obese fifty-year old, I spent thirty-five years in quiet agony, with my weight bouncing up and down between 135 pounds and 220 pounds, a range of 85 pounds. Over and over again. I am 5'5" tall, so you can see that I was heavy for my height.

I tried nearly every weight loss program available, from daily visits to the fat doctor to Optifast liquid diets to Weight Watchers, Jenny Craig, Atkins and more. Many more.

And, I was wildly successful at taking off weight. Just like Oprah, I gloried in my skinny jeans after a liquid diet. I lost 60 pounds after the birth of my second child on a starvation, 600 calorie per day diet and kept it off for maybe.....60 days. I ate grapefruit on the South Beach diet, packaged food purchased on visits to Jenny Craig and lost about 20 pounds on both of these programs—which came right back as soon as I stopped.

I've taken diet pills, both prescription and over-the-counter. I've had liposuction on my thighs and butt. Uh oh...that was a secret until now. I've joined a gym and never used my membership. I've been to fat farms... err...spas...for cucumber fasts and cleansing massages. I've gone to therapists, weight loss counselors and hypnosis specialists to be hypnotized to not crave ice cream. Actually, I liked the hypnosis because it worked!

You could say that I am a very experienced consumer of weight loss programs.

But, until I decided to change my daily habits, I was not successful at weight control.

And then, one day, my father dropped dead from a heart attack

There were no signs that my father had heart disease. And he was a doctor! On a sunny Monday in June, he had a heart attack in his medical office and drove himself home so he wouldn't scare his patients. He collapsed at home, in front of my mother, which of course, terrified her.

My grandfather, his father, had also died from a sudden heart attack, at a much younger age than my father. So there it was, the shocking, irrefutable proof that heart disease runs in my family and I might be next. I was 45 years old, obese with lousy eating habits, stressed at work, stressed as a busy mother at home, and taking better care of the family dog than I was of myself.

Clearly, something had to change. I didn't want to die young.

Five years of trial and error, research, commitment and practicing new habits

My lifestyle of bad eating habits didn't change overnight. Plus, it was really hard to let go of hoping for a quick cure, finding that miracle diet which would change my world, melting pounds away and "give me the body I've always wanted". It's embarrassing to admit that I actually believed this nonsense for so many years.

Diets are for short-term goals with short-term results. Weight control habits support long-term goals with long-term results.

I hated having to accept this. I really wanted a short-term miracle diet to work for the rest of my life. When I finally, truly understood that I needed to find another way, it was like being cast out into the wilderness with no map, no compass and no way to find shelter. But I knew I had to learn a new direction. For five years, I read every book I could find, took classes, talked to nutritionists, doctors, therapists, personal trainers and anyone I thought who could help. I researched nutrition, effective exercises and ways to control cravings. I was willing to try many new things, but what I was <u>not</u> willing to do was abandon my commitment to keeping extra pounds off. I had unshakeable faith that I could learn to maintain my weight at a healthy level.

Are you ready to make this commitment? If you are, you can absolutely believe that you will learn how to control your weight, too!

Weight Control That Works: 10 Daily Habits can be your map, your guidebook to a new, healthy lifestyle.

Sharing how I mastered weight control

I'm qualified to write this book because I have first-hand experience with the challenges of managing weight. Weight control is not an academic research topic for me. I have lived it. After 35 years of being overweight, punctuated by yo-yo diets, I finally learned to control my weight and lost 85 pounds, which have successfully stayed off for 18 years. Yes, that's a grand total of 53 years of experience. It's wonderful to be a slender, healthy older woman knowing that I have mastered one of modern life's most difficult skills.

This makes me someone with wisdom to share.

You can learn from people who are successful at achieving your same goal, especially those who are older and more experienced. You can save time, money, effort and...yes...heartbreak by gathering knowledge from other people who have dealt successfully with your same challenges.

- I know what it feels like to have a craving and not be able to stop stuffing food in my mouth. When I say that something has worked to control cravings, you can believe me.

- I know what it feels like to be a post-menopausal woman, to be frightened about the changes in my body and overwhelmed by knowing that I will have to make major changes to stay healthy.

- I know what it feels like to be a younger woman, resentful that my heavy appearance made such a difference in how people judged me. I understand the emotional roller coaster that comes with being obese in our culture.

- I know what it feels like to have my thighs rub together and make a rash. I know too well being filled with shame about my body, then needing to be brave and carry on every day.

- I know what it feels like to be on a controlled diet and have friends be loud in their support, then silent as I got fat again.

And...I know the unbelievable relief of finally mastering my eating and weight issues so I can take that enormous amount of attention and emotion my overweight body used to demand and apply these to a happier, more creative life!

My goal is to make your journey towards mastering weight control easier

This book is packed with practical advice about how you can master controlling your weight, take off the extra pounds and finally be relaxed with your body. You can do this at any age.

For those of you who are younger, you are so lucky to be building healthy life-style habits early, and avoid being as uncomfortable in your thirties and forties as I was. Congratulations for being smart about planning for your future.

For those readers who are menopausal or older, there is hope! You deserve applause for continuing to improve your life. Never give up! Certainly it's a challenge to control our weight as we age, but you can absolutely do it! I'm living proof.

Women helping other women

Writing a book takes time and effort, and how-to books often function like big business cards, explaining what the author has to offer so you'll buy it. Please know that *I have no financial investments in any diet products or clinics. I'm not a weight loss professional looking for clients.*

So, why would I go to the effort of writing a book?

It's all about leaving a positive legacy. Like many women in their sixties, I feel a strong urge to help other people. My children are grown but I still love teaching what I've learned about the world. Teaching others is the greatest opportunity to stay focused and continue to learn. Many older women become volunteers in their community. I do that, and I also write books about how women can reinvent their lives.

This is my first book about weight control and body image. It's been a deeply private subject for me and it wasn't easy to open up about how desperate I was to find a better way to live with my body.

Over the years, many friends have urged me to share how I was able to turn my life around because they were inspired by my example, but I always resisted. I was shy about stepping forward and saying "This works!".

But my attitude has changed. These days I'm dismayed about the obesity epidemic. And I know first-hand that so many women are deeply unhappy with their bodies and heading towards years of health problems.

If what I've learned about controlling my weight and restoring my health can help make your life better, the effort to write this book is worth it.

I would love to hear about your challenges and successes. Please email me at Christie@HopefulWoman.com

Now...let's look at how you can control your weight and change your life.

HOW TO USE THIS BOOK

Weight Control That Works is your road map to sustainable weight control.

It's about learning to move past the wishful thinking that quick-fix diets offer. You cannot lose 20 pounds in 20 days and hope to keep them off. Sadly, there are no miracle products that will melt belly fat. You know this! If you have opened this book, you're thinking that it's time to be realistic and practical. It's time for you to take action for long-term, positive results.

Anyone can hop on a fad diet and take off a few pounds in the short-term. But only someone committed to good health and willing to make lifestyle changes will be able to take off weight and *keep it off.*

We've all heard the statement "Diets don't work" but actually accepting this and knowing that it's time to change your habits for long-term results is a big shift.

Congratulations on being ready!

Why lifestyle habits are different than a weight loss diet

One of the many reasons why weight loss diets don't work is because a diet is an intervention in your normal life. When you stop the program and go back to what you usually do, the pounds come back.

So, the answer is obvious, isn't it? *You need to change your lifestyle.* Your normal daily life needs to support losing weight and keeping it off. The 10 Daily Habits will give you guidance about how to do this.

Practicing and then absorbing these habits so they are simply your normal behavior is how you will get off the yo-yo diet merry-go-round.

Say goodbye to temporary interventions. What you will be learning is a long-term lifestyle, supported by good behavior and good nutrition for good health. Yes, that's three goods!

Here's where to begin.

PART ONE: START BY LEARNING WHY YOU ARE UNIQUE

There are millions of people who are overweight but you have a unique story. Part One explains why this is true. Only you have your own unique combination of genetic inheritance, metabolism, childhood training, and current lifestyle.

Part One will walk you through these four elements so you can have a deeper understanding and be more motivated to make the necessary changes for your weight control success.

PART TWO: 10 DAILY HABITS FOR WEIGHT CONTROL THAT WORKS

Each of the *10 Daily Habits* has its own chapter with a description of what to do and why it's a healthy, long-term choice.

The habits are listed from the start of your day, beginning with *Habit #1: Get Enough Sleep.* While you can read the habits in any order, you will need <u>all of them</u> to successfully control your weight permanently. But, if you prefer, you can skip around when reading.

As a long-time dieter, you are probably familiar with some of the material, like the call to exercise 30 minutes every day. *(Habit #3: Exercise for 30 Minutes Every Day.)* But, don't skip that chapter! I have years of experience keeping extra pounds off, and just may have something new to tell you!

Be sure to carefully read and reread any chapters that are new concepts to you. They are packed with valuable information and useful tips to make learning each habit easier.

18

PART THREE: THE 4 WEEK PROGRAM TO LEARN THE 10 DAILY HABITS

Part Three outlines a four-week program that will help you integrate the 10 Daily Habits into your lifestyle.

If you think that learning ten new habits at once is a lot to absorb, you're right! *Part Three* breaks this down so you can comfortably learn a select number of new behaviors each week. When those behaviors become second nature, they are habits.

Learning new habits doesn't happen overnight, but you will find that it doesn't take long to shift your behavior if you are truly committed to weight control. You will soon feel comfortable with your new lifestyle choices, and reinforced by your weight control success.

There is no motivation as powerful as happiness and success.

PART FOUR: 4 BONUS HABITS

Part Four includes four valuable bonus habits that will help you develop a healthy lifestyle and control your weight. They are especially useful during your period of transition from a lifestyle that promotes weight gain to a lifestyle that supports maintaining your body weight at a healthy level.

The 4 Bonus Habits are easy to learn. You are probably familiar with one of them: *Bonus Habit #2: Keep a Food Diary*. The others are particularly valuable for managing a transition to a new way of eating. Having specific actions you can repeat during the transition period will help keep you on track.

Be sure to read all 4 Bonus Habits as you start planning how to manage your day-to-day life with the commitment to sustainable weight control.

PART FIVE: RESOURCES FOR LEARNING MORE

When it comes to weight control, curiosity is your best friend! It's easier to stay motivated if you are surrounded by the voices of people who share your goals for healthy living.

Part Five: Resources for Learning More is a list of books, videos, websites and apps I recommend from my personal experience as useful to learn more about healthy habits. *Most of these did not exist twenty years ago.* Back then, I was blindly feeling my way, learning by trial and error which habits would control my weight and be comfortable to live with everyday. Thank goodness these resources are available now.

You will also learn more about an endless fascinating topic: how your body works.

Be a life-long learner for a longer life!

AS ALWAYS, CHECK WITH YOUR DOCTOR BEFORE YOU START

Consider showing this book to your doctor so s/he can look at the table of contents. It's important that you feel confident about doing the right thing for your metabolism and overall health, and your doctor agrees.

When preparing to write *Weight Control That Works*, I consulted with numerous doctors including bariatric specialists who run weight loss clinics, pediatricians who work with childhood obesity, and internists. Two experienced nutritionists also gave me valuable feedback while I was developing how the information from my research and personal experience would be presented. Medical and nutrition consultants helped confirm the accuracy of what I've written in the book.

And, I encourage you to do your own research! Knowledge is power.

NO FAT SHAMING OR FEAR

This book is not about motivation through fear or shame. As someone who struggled with being obese, I know too well the discomfort of being fat shamed. It's a very humiliating experience. So, let me be clear, this book is not about appearances. It's about maintaining our health as we grow older by maintaining a healthy lifestyle and a healthy weight for our height.

You can improve the prospects for your longterm health by taking good care of your body. You need knowledge about what to do and you need compassion for yourself. Don't beat yourself up that you have weight to lose. Don't waste energy on guilt and shame. Just get on with the business of taking care of yourself.

THE BMI CHART FOR REFERENCE: FIND YOUR BODY MASS INDEX

The easiest way to find out if your weight is proportional and healthy for your height is to find your place on the Body Mass Index Chart. Look down the left side for your height, then across for your weight. Up at the top will be your BMI ranking. Down at the bottom, you'll see if you fall into one of the following three categories: Healthy Weight, Overweight and Obese.

When I started researching the 10 Daily Habits for Weight Control almost 20 years ago, I weighed 220 pounds at 5'5" tall. My BMI was off the chart! Over 35! I was not only obese, I was what doctors call "morbidly obese". At 45 years old, it was clearly time to change my lifestyle. Today, I am 135 pounds, still 5'5" tall, and my BMI is between 22 and 23, within the range of healthy weight.

Find your BMI with this chart:

BMI	19	20	21	22	23	24	25	26	27	28	29	30	31	32	33	34	35

Height: Weight in Pounds

Height	19	20	21	22	23	24	25	26	27	28	29	30	31	32	33	34	35
5'0"	97	102	107	112	118	123	128	133	138	143	148	153	158	163	168	174	179
5'1"	100	106	111	116	122	127	132	137	143	148	153	158	164	169	174	180	185
5'2"	104	109	115	120	126	131	136	142	147	153	158	164	169	175	180	186	191
5'3"	107	113	118	124	130	135	141	146	152	158	163	169	175	180	186	191	197
5'4"	110	116	122	128	134	140	145	151	157	163	169	174	180	186	192	197	204
5'5"	114	120	123	132	138	144	150	156	162	168	174	180	186	192	198	204	210
5'6"	118	124	130	136	142	148	155	161	167	173	179	186	192	198	204	210	216
5'7"	121	127	134	140	146	153	159	166	172	178	185	191	198	204	211	217	223
5'8"	125	131	138	144	151	158	164	171	177	184	190	197	203	210	216	223	230
5'9"	128	135	142	149	155	162	169	176	182	189	196	203	209	216	223	230	236
5'10"	132	139	146	153	160	167	174	181	188	195	202	209	216	222	229	236	243
5'11"	136	143	150	157	165	172	179	186	193	200	208	215	222	229	236	243	250
6'0"	140	147	154	162	169	177	184	191	199	206	213	221	228	235	242	250	258

Healthy Weight   Overweight   Obese

Here is an online BMI calculator from Harvard Health Publications from the Harvard Medical School:

http://www.health.harvard.edu/diet-and-weight-loss/bmi-calculator

According to the Harvard Medical School, your BMI matters if your number is high as it indicates your higher risk of developing diabetes, arthritis, liver disease, several types of cancer (including those of breast, colon and prostate), high blood pressure, high cholesterol and sleep apnea.

So…losing weight and keeping it off is not about fitting into your skinny jeans, although that's good, too. Who doesn't love looking great and hearing compliments? But, there's more to a long, healthy life than whether your clothes fit. Changing to a weight control lifestyle is about protecting yourself from the health risks of obesity.

YOU CAN DO THIS!

Shifting from worrying about what to do into a commitment to take action will make you feel better. Instantly. You know you will be working towards positive change.

The time is now. You have the road map in your hands to learn and change your life.

PART ONE

START BY LEARNING
WHY YOU ARE UNIQUE

**There is no one exactly like you.
Only you have your unique combination
of genetic heritage, metabolism,
childhood training and current lifestyle.**

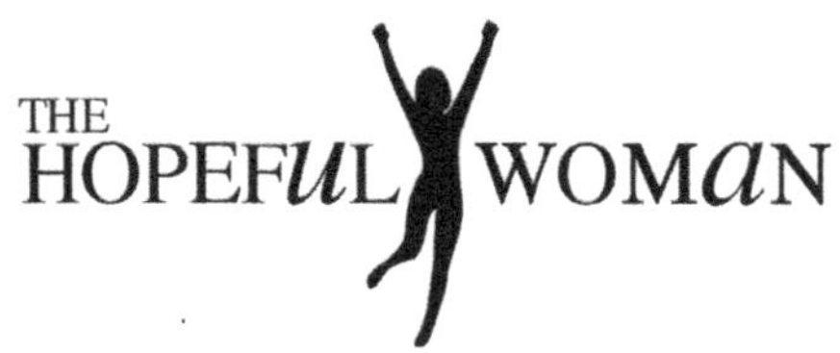

THERE IS NO ONE EXACTLY LIKE YOU

There are millions of people who are overweight today and each one has a unique story. Everyone has a unique combination of genetic inheritance, metabolism, childhood training and current lifestyle.

With so many people wanting to lose weight, how can I know for certain that you are truly unique and one of a kind? It's because your individual life has blended four factors together in ways that no one else shares. Not one single person alive or dead has ever blended these four factors in exactly the same way as you.

The four factors for your unique blend are:

- Your family's genetic gifts: Your health inheritance.

- Your current metabolism: How all your internal systems are working.

- Childhood training: What you ate as a child. Favorite foods are an acquired taste.

- Your current lifestyle: Your eating, drinking, exercise, sleep and spending habits as you currently live day to day.

Each of these four factors has an immensely strong influence on whether you have been able to control your weight as an adult. Two are unchangeable: your genetic inheritance and your childhood training. The other two factors are either within your control or ability to get help: improving how your metabolism functions, and your daily lifestyle of eating, drinking, exercise, sleep and spending.

There is another factor—your willingness to make permanent changes for weight control—but we'll get to that along the way.

Let's take a closer look at all four factors and what they each mean for you.

YOUR FAMILY'S GENETIC GIFTS: YOUR HEALTH INHERITANCE

There is much we inherit from our parents besides the color of our hair, skin and general appearance. Unlike what we easily see on the outside, our metabolic health inheritance can be something of a mystery, but you have probably heard that certain types of cancer, heart disease, high blood pressure and high cholesterol can run in families.

Inside and outside, you are a unique mix of your parents' genetic gifts. Unless we have a metabolic disorder diagnosed in childhood, most of us don't think very much about our genetic inheritance until we are older or there is a health crisis in our lives.

That certainly describes me. I was lucky to have grown up without significant illness and even though my weight went wildly up and down, I wasn't paying much attention to what was going on inside my body until my father suddenly died.

My father dropped dead from a heart attack

My father quite unexpectedly had a massive heart attack one day and died. We were all caught by surprise.

I was forty-five years old when he died, and I was just beginning to notice aging issues. Up to that day, I could have told you many significant numbers—my shoe size, my weight, my salary—but I didn't know my blood pressure numbers, or any other medically significant number. I went to regular check-ups and the doctor would say "Christie, you should lose some weight" and I would go on a crash diet, drop pounds, then gain everything back.

Basically, I only cared about what I could see in the mirror. I took my insides for granted.

My grandfather, my father's father, had also died from a sudden a heart attack. He was quite young, only fifty-five. So, there it was: it seemed irrefutable that heart disease runs in my family. The shock of my dad's death made me realize I'd better start paying attention to my long-term health. My usual behavior of yo-yo diets, irregular eating habits and sporadic exercise wasn't being responsible or taking good care of my heart….or my morale.

It often takes a shock in your life to be the catalyst for change. Just hearing about health risks in the abstract doesn't seem to be enough. We live in denial or hope and keep up our bad habits, thinking that there will be time to catch up, or somebody will invent a Magic Pill to make any problems go away.

With a family history of heart disease, and the fact that my next big birthday was The Big Five Oh, my father's sudden death was the event that changed my attitude profoundly. The day my father died was the day that I committed to learning about my metabolism, paying attention to my long-term health and changing my habits.

Not everyone can know their family's medical history. But, if you are fortunate to know the health histories of both sides of your family, especially high blood pressure, high cholesterol, diabetes and heart disease, you have good reasons to be paying attention by getting regular doctor checkups and living a healthy life-style.

YOUR METABOLISM:
HOW YOUR INTERNAL SYSTEMS ARE WORKING

Let's take a very quick look at what goes on inside your body.

Your metabolism is a complex set of chemical reactions that your body needs to stay alive. Basic energy production is a metabolic function: your enzymes are breaking down food so your body can use it for fuel right away or store the components for use later. This is how we make extra fat! We eat more than our bodies need to use for immediate fuel at our current activity level.

To work well, your metabolism needs foods that are high in nutrients but many of us eat foods that are "empty calories". In other words, we eat sugars and extra fats our bodies don't need. We are not getting the proteins, vitamins, minerals and fibers we do need if most of our calories do not come from fresh vegetables, lean proteins, whole fruits and whole grains.

You may have heard the expression: "You get the first thirty years for free, after that, you get the body you deserve." It seems a little harsh but it's a way of saying that we can get away with things when we are young. Things like eating lots of desserts, junk, drinking too much, skipping meals and hitting the vending machines at work. Or not having an exercise plan. No worries, some people in their 20's say, I'll do the South Beach and drop those pounds by summer.

When you're over thirty, it just gets harder. And over fifty, much harder. It's perfectly understandable to be in denial. Who wants to admit that they're growing older and their body needs more care and attention? Isn't it bad enough that advertisers tell us to be worried about wrinkles and gray hair, but now we have to take care of our blood pressure, cholesterol and blood sugar too?! We can't even see these things!

If I spend an afternoon getting a new hairstyle, it's immediately good and I'll see the difference. For me, it was a tough transition from being a young woman who only needed to worry about how I looked to being a middle-aged woman with potentially health-threatening consequences from being obese. My father's death was a real wake-up call for me.

In this book, we are going to discuss many aspects of metabolism. I hope you find them to be as interesting as I do. I love learning how things work. And what could be more vital than learning about our bodies?

YOUR CHILDHOOD TRAINING: TASTES YOU LEARNED TO LOVE EARLY ARE HARD TO CHANGE

Our preferences for what tastes good and foods we like to eat are set very early in childhood. As a young child, you were capable of learning to like or dislike a wide variety of foods and, certainly, what you were offered made a big difference in shaping your preferences today.

A baby is born able to taste sweet foods and has a natural predisposition to reject foods that taste bitter or sour. The taste of salt develops at about four months. Babies also learn quickly which foods sit comfortably in their stomachs and which foods make them feel uncomfortable. Researchers think that high-fat foods make babies feel full and satisfied. You can see that the tastes for high-sugar, high-fat, high-salt foods can develop very early.

The human tongue has between two and ten thousand taste buds

Did you know that these amazing sensory receptors are replaced every two weeks? (Did you even notice your taste buds being replaced? I never have!) We have more taste buds when we're young than at any other time in our lives. Older adults are said to have lost fifty-percent of their taste buds, which is why food can taste bland to them. Thanks to their abundance of taste buds, children can have a very acute sense of taste and can develop very intense food preferences.

Taste is a composite sense, of course—your nose is heavily involved, both in anticipating the taste of food when you smell its aroma and also when you chew, sending chemicals up your nasal passages. The sense of smell also works best when people are young.

If you haven't been offered a diet of fresh vegetables, fresh fruits and whole grains as a child, you may have some re-learning to do overcoming your childhood food preferences. In the United States, there are many families who have raised their children on fast and processed food, especially over the last thirty years. If this is what you ate as a child, you probably love it.

My mother served broiled chicken frequently, along with ample portions of green vegetables and a salad with every dinner. I was lucky that way. Today, chicken is my favorite meat and I love salads. My Chinese friends have their preferences based on the foods their families cooked. One of my German friends wants bread and butter with each meal, and ends every dinner with a sweet dessert because that's the way he grew up.

If you were raised on a high-sugar, high-fat, high-salt diet, it can be very difficult to unlearn these preferences, even when you recognize that continuing to eat this way is unhealthy.

Food preferences are different than taste preferences.

A "food preference" is the selection of one food over another. Cuisines around the world have different materials to work with and different cultures have been amazingly inventive in creating foods that are now considered traditional. Ten different people may love sweet food, but, depending on their backgrounds, they may make ten different choices about which sweet food to eat.

A "taste preference" is favoring one flavor over another out of the five basic choices our sense of taste gives us: sweet, sour, bitter, salty and umami (savory). Some people have a natural sweet tooth that persists their whole lives. Other folks develop to prefer salty food. Personally, I really dislike sour and bitter food so avoid these tastes, but my youngest son loves sour. As a child, the sour candies were always his first choice, to my amazement!

Give some thought to how
you were trained to eat as a child.

Remembering how you were trained to eat as a child, and thinking about how your food preferences were originally formed will make a big difference when you try to form new food preferences in the future.

If you have trouble staying attracted to healthy eating habits, it might be because the pull of childhood food preferences is so strong. Children often resist eating unfamiliar foods and this resistance to change can carry over into adulthood.

So, if you like what you like and don't want to change, that's completely normal!

But....if you are going to control your weight....being willing to consider learning new food preferences will be important. It won't happen overnight, but you can learn to love and appreciate different foods. And no one is saying that you can never have your old favorite foods.

If they're high-fat, high-sugar, just make them occasional treats, not everyday meals.

What is food neophobia?

Did you know that the refusal to try new foods actually has a name? It's called "Food Neophobia" and it's the subject of many serious studies as researchers are trying to learn why people, children especially, refuse to try new foods.

Food neophobia is seen across all cultures and often persists into adulthood. It's different than being a picky eater. Picky eaters will find reasons to reject familiar as well as unfamiliar foods but someone with food neophobia rejects only unfamiliar food.

If you are unwilling to try new foods, you may hold yourself back from being able to master weight control. For example, if you grew up eating fried foods, pizza and sweets, you may constantly turn your nose up at salads and fresh vegetables.

You can learn to love different food choices:
Taste new food at least 15 times.

So, what can you do if you want to change to a more healthy diet but you hate vegetables unless they're smothered in cheese? Or, you love to load your coffee with sweetener. The good news is that repeated exposure can shift your opinion and YOU CAN LEARN TO LOVE NEW FOOD.

The magic number is fifteen. Researchers have found that, on average, someone needs to taste a new food at least fifteen times before that food starts to taste good, especially if you have a built-in preference for old tastes.

Let's take coffee with sweetener as an example. If you prefer your coffee loaded with sugar or sweetener, you may find plain coffee to be dull, even repulsive. I had to force myself to drink coffee without any sweetener for weeks before I started preferring it this way. Yes, it finally worked!

Here's another example: I used to put a lot of salad dressing on my green salads. Then, I moved to "dressing on the side" when I order at restaurants. At home, I stopped using dressing entirely by increasing the variety of toppings on salads. The months went by and now I'm so used to eating green salads without any dressing that having an oily or sweet coating on everything tastes wrong to me. I truly prefer my salads dry and clean. (And...I save hundreds of calories this way!)

YOUR CURRENT LIFESTYLE: YOUR SLEEPING, EATING & DRINKING AND EXERCISE HABITS

After your inherited metabolism, nothing has greater impact on your longterm health and ability to feel good than your daily sleeping, eating, drinking and exercise habits. Your family may have taught you habits, or you may have fallen into habits over the years of doing your best to get through the day.

To control your weight, you need to be honest and clear-sighted about your normal daily habits. Being observant about your daily life is the best starting place for making positive change. It may seem overwhelming to change your sleep, eating, drinking and exercise habits all at once. Don't do that. You'll find advice about how to incorporate new healthy habits into your life in *Part Three: The 4 Week Program for Learning the 10 Daily Habits.*

In the meantime, let's take a quick look at the major lifestyle influences on your weight. They will be covered in much more detail in the following chapters.

Sleep: Are you sleep deprived? Do you need to eat to have more energy? Are you unable to resist food temptations?

When I first started writing this book and talked with friends about the importance of sleep for weight control, most people were very surprised. They had never considered the role that sleep plays in helping your body—especially your brain—reset itself to be able to deal with the stresses and challenges of each day.

Sleep is so important for weight control that I made it *Habit #1: Get Enough Sleep.*

Both your willpower and your appetite are affected by lack of sleep. So, if you typically get less sleep than your body needs (and most people need seven hours) you can expect it will be harder to control both your eating and your weight.

Eating and drinking:
The most obvious lifestyle components
of weight control

If you have lost weight on an intervention diet and have gained the weight back, and now you want to change this pattern, it's time to seriously look at the food you eat in your everyday life. You owe it to yourself to have more knowledge and to be able to make informed decisions.

You need to know what happens when you eat and drink. Where does the sugar go? What does it do? Why is refined white flour treated like sugar by your body? Just why is everyone screaming at you to eat whole grains?

Everyone understands that if you eat too much, you will gain weight. But, not everyone understands that you can eat enormous amounts of food and not gain any weight if you chose high fiber, low sugar, low fat foods. This includes most vegetables, whole grains, legumes, many fruits and lean meats.

Six out of ten habits in this book directly address eating and drinking lifestyle habits. And not just what and how much you are eating. *When* you eat is important, too. For example, starting the day with protein is a far superior choice to starting the day with a donut. (A donut is fried refined white flour coated with sugar. Sure, it tastes good, but it will reek havoc on your ability to sustain your energy for the morning.)

There is so much more to say and learn here about eating and drinking. Whole university departments are devoted to nutrition and biochemistry. This book can't possibly cover it all, but I've done my best to share with you the crucial points anyone trying to control their weight needs to know.

And don't forget, our understanding of how the human body works is expanding all the time. There is a constant stream of new knowledge.

Keep learning! Just watch out for the quacks. Pick your information from people who rely on science and common sense.

If the seller of a diet program tells you that you can have it all by eating pizza and chocolate, run the other way!

It takes practice to create a healthy relationship with food

Be patient and kind with yourself. It's not easy to move away from processed foods, sugar, sweets and all the goodies being advertised all around you. Caring about your long term health more than immediate taste pleasure takes courage and commitment.

I promise you that the future is also very pleasurable. Once you have learned to love healthy, whole foods in smaller portions you will enjoy eating and will feel as good as you look.

Exercise: Your body was born to move. It likes it!

There is no magic bullet for good health that comes close to regular, daily exercise. For weight control, no drug you can buy over the counter or from your pharmacist will come close to the benefits your body derives from being moved. Walking, stretching, swimming, bending....it's all very, very good.

Unless your career keeps you on the move physically, you need to schedule regular movement into your day to be able to control your weight. And the movement doesn't need to be a huge gym workout. Walking and fidgeting will help tremendously. Are you sitting in a chair reading this right now? Squeeze your butt! Flex your abs! Tense your thighs! Wiggle your feet! You could be fidgeting right now.

There is only one chapter on exercise in this book because the benefits are so obvious and it's so well known. You probably know everything in this chapter already. Fair enough, but skim it just to make sure. You might just learn something new. See *Habit #3: Exercise for 30 Minutes Every Day.*

CONGRATULATIONS! YOU DESERVE CREDIT FOR LEARNING ABOUT A NEW LIFESTYLE

Since you are reading this book, you understand that continuing to diet and gain weight back is a pattern that is not working for you. You understand that you need to try something different. It's not an easy decision. The temptations to hop on another weight loss diet program are all around us. On the television, in the supermarket, in so many magazines, you are bombarded by weight loss promises if you only sign up for their program.

But, again, a weight loss program is an intervention into your normal, daily lifestyle. It works because it interrupts what you usually do when you're on your own. When it ends, you're on your own again….with no advice about how to structure your daily life for optimal weight control.

Now, you have *Weight Control That Works: 10 Daily Habits to Take Weight Off, Keep it Off and Love Your Body.* Read this book and you will know what to do to control your weight. For life.

New behaviors become old habits surprisingly quickly!

Humans are by nature highly adaptable. Look at how we've migrated all over the world, living in different environments from ice fields to jungles. In the 21st century, we're having to adapt again, to an environment of fast food, endless advertisements, desk jobs and incredibly busy, stressful lives.

Never forget that you can do this! I hope that understanding how you are truly unique and one of a kind will help you get started.

PART TWO

10 DAILY HABITS FOR
WEIGHT CONTROL THAT WORKS

**Why have just a short period of weight loss
when you can keep the weight off for life?**

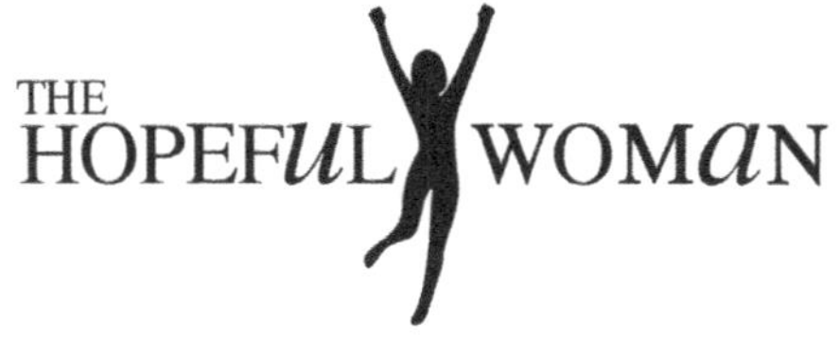

HABIT #1
GET ENOUGH SLEEP

**Willpower and appetite
are affected by sleep deprivation.
Getting enough sleep is critical for weight control.**

Did you know that lack of sleep directly influences your willpower? It's not just a matter of being tired and reaching for a sugary snack for energy. *Not getting enough sleep alters the hormonal balance in your body.*

You know that hormones have direct influence on behavior. Hormones can drive teenagers crazy, help new mothers bond to their infants, cause a fight or flight response. Hormones also have a direct influence on your appetite. And, when you don't get enough sleep, those hormones are thrown out of balance.

The consequences are enormous. Your brain's ability to regulate your appetite and tell you when you're hungry and when to stop eating is just one of the negative results. You lose your willpower when faced with urgent hunger. Even worse, the hormones that control how your cells absorb energy in the form of glucose are also affected. We are going to take a closer look at both of these hormonal responses to sleep deprivation in the pages that follow.

Yes, it's generally bad news. There is no way to describe lack of enough sleep as a healthy choice for weight control. In fact, it's a powerful negative force that will sabotage your best efforts.

Most diets don't address sleep as a vital component. Since this book is about longterm weight control and not short-term weight loss, you must be aware how your full day's activities—all 24 hours—influence your ability to control your weight.

How much sleep do you actually need?

Most people require seven to eight hours a night for their metabolism to function at optimal levels. In today's stressed, busy world, that's unrealistic for many of us. Are you working two jobs and raising a family? Do you have a new baby? When I was working and raising children, getting five hours a night was a major achievement.

The good news is that it takes very few nights of full sleep to restore your hormonal balance. That's why so many people try to "bank" sleep on the weekend. It really does help. Naps help, too. Sometimes we're just stuck in circumstances we must live through, but if there's any way you can get more sleep you will see immediate benefits with increased energy, a faster metabolism and more willpower.

Do everything you possibly can to protect your sleep time!

If you have trouble going to bed because of distractions like TV or the Internet, remember being tired means you have less willpower to resist. That means resisting anything. Distractions are more powerful when you're tired. Turn off your TV and your computer and go to bed!

You simply need enough sleep to be able to control your weight.

Let's look at why.

Sleep and willpower:
Here's how lack of sleep sabotages your self-control.

You know that drinking and drugs influence the functioning of your brain, but did you know that lack of sleep affects your brain just like being slightly drunk? <u>Judgment and self-control are diminished when you're sleep deprived</u>, just like when you've had too much to drink.

Self-control is a complex interaction between behavior centers in your prefrontal cortex—the front part of your brain which is in charge of executive function. Scientists mapping and matching behavior to brain regions have found three specific areas in the prefrontal cortex that work together to create will-power and self-control. It's these three areas that organize goals and desires, make you feel responsible and keep you on task. Sleep deprivation affects the prefrontal cortex's ability to keep these areas working smoothly.

So, your capacity for impulse control is reduced when your brain can't function a peak performance due to lack of sleep. It becomes more difficult to resist temptations. Cravings can grow and call to you. You act impulsively and grab foods that are loaded with added sugar because you're tired and want more energy.

For longterm weight control, not having optimal impulse control is an obviously dangerous situation. Being chronically sleep deprived—getting less than six hours of sleep a night—is a fast way to sabotage your willpower and self-control.

The good news is that this is reversible! With just a few nights of solid, uninterrupted sleep, you can give your brain the rest it needs. Your prefrontal cortex will recover and be able to function at its best.

But the story of weight control and sleep is a complicated one. Hormones make a difference, too.

Let's take a look.

Sleep affects your hormones ghrelin and leptin.
Hormones affect appetite.
Lack of sleep makes your appetite grow.

Sleep deprivation is a form of physical stress with multiple consequences. An important one is that your hormones are influenced directly by how much sleep you get. Two key regulatory hormones, ghrelin and leptin, need to work in balance to control your appetite, but lack of sleep alters their production and throws off their balance.

You can profoundly change your body's ability to manage your appetite by not sleeping. Here's how:

- Ghrelin is the hormone that stimulates your appetite so you feel like eating. When you don't get enough sleep, your brain signals the release of more ghrelin so you want to eat more.

- The ghrelin hormone is primarily secreted by the lining of the stomach. Normally, your stomach makes ghrelin when it's empty, but lack of sleep disrupts the cycle, possibly as a reaction to needing more energy to keep functioning for more hours. Less sleep equals more ghrelin circulating in your system resulting in your brain urging you to eat more.

- Leptin is the hormone that suppresses your appetite and tells you that you're no longer hungry. If you're sleep deprived, less leptin is released so your brain doesn't give you the message to stop eating.

- The leptin hormone is secreted primarily by fat cells. (Surprise! Fat cells are not passive.) Less sleep equals less leptin available in your system which results in your brain not knowing when to stop eating.

Lack of sleep makes your hunger grow and reduces your sense of fullness and satisfaction when you do eat. The result is you eat more.

Both ghrelin and leptin act on your brain via the hypothalamus, the immensely powerful brain region that regulates hormone production throughout the body. When your brain is functioning properly, normal feelings of hunger are controlled by switching ghrelin and leptin on and off.

Regretfully, it doesn't take too many days of missing sleep to negatively affect the functioning of your hypothalamus. Many studies have proven that after just a few nights of restricted sleep, the average human brain loses its capacity to control appetite.

Are people who sleep fewer hours fatter?

A study at Stanford University gathered data from 1,024 people.* They reported how many hours of sleep each person got per night and charted the participants' levels of leptin and ghrelin. Then, their weights were measured.

<u>People who slept less than eight hours each night had more body fat</u>. Their levels of leptin were lower and their levels of ghrelin were higher. There was a direct correlation between sleep and body fat: *The people in the study who slept the least also weighed the most.*

If you take nothing else away from this book, let it be that you need a solid night's sleep in order to control your weight.

When people challenge me to tell them something new about losing weight and keeping it off, they are always surprised when the first thing I say is: *You must get enough sleep.* We are so programmed to think that our weight is only determined by what we eat and how much we exercise, but that's hardly the whole picture. Our bodies are complex systems with dynamic and complicated parts which work together to great a healthy whole. If you deny your body the sleep it needs, there will be physical consequences.

Do everything possible to protect your sleeping hours for optimal success at weight control.

Short Sleep Duration Is Associated with Reduced Leptin, Elevated Gherlin, and Increased Body Mass Index by Shahrad Taheri, Ling Lin, Diane Austin, Terry Young, Emmanuel Mignot. Published December 7, 2004, Public Library of Science. For more information about the Stanford sleep studies, see The Stanford Center for Sleep Sciences and Medicine. www.sleep.stanford.edu

Sleep apnea and obesity

The National Sleep Foundation estimates that 18 million Americans have sleep apnea.

Sleep apnea is a breathing disorder caused by compromised respiratory function. In other words, it's a blockage of the nose and throat. Apnea is often associated with weight gain across the neck and top of the body. If you sleep alone, you may not be aware that you have apnea, except for feeling very tired during the day. If you have a sleep partner, listen to what s/he has to say about your breathing.

Sleep apnea and obesity are a cycle. You feel tired so you are less inclined to exercise. You are more inclined to eat high sugar carbohydrates for energy. You gain more weight. You sleep more poorly.

If you know or think you have sleep apnea, ask your doctor for a referral to a sleep clinic. It's quite well established that losing weight has a significant, positive effect on improving sleep apnea by helping to remove the obstructions and pressure on your respiratory system.

Why you need to know more about the hormone leptin

Other hormones are more famous. Testosterone, for example. Leptin is possibly the most powerful hormone unknown by the general public. It wasn't discovered until 1994. I was already 47 years old by then, and had gained and lost the same 85 pounds without giving my hormones a single thought! But since 1994, leptin's role in human metabolism has been studied extensively.

Here is more information about what leptin does and why lack of sleep makes a difference:

- Leptin is made in your fat cells and travels in your bloodstream to the hypothalamus, the part of your brain that regulates all hormones. Leptin levels signal your brain about required food intake, how much energy to spend and how much energy to store. (Fat cells are your body's energy storage system.) If your leptin signal is working properly, you have a normal appetite, can produce enough energy to burn fat, feel healthy and keep your weight at a stable level.

- When your leptin signals are too low, the brain thinks you're starving. It cuts your energy level so you feel tired and lazy. It stimulates your appetite.

- If your leptin levels are high enough, the hypothalamus signals that you feel full and satisfied. You stop eating. You can, however, develop leptin resistance, which means that your hypothalamus never receives the "satisfied" message and you continue to eat.

- Leptin interacts with signals to release insulin. Low leptin levels cause the brain to stimulate more insulin release, which drives more energy into your fat cells.

Put very simply: low leptin levels mean less energy for activity, more hunger and more fat cells being formed.

- Lack of sleep suppresses the production of leptin. People with sleep apnea also show low leptin levels because their sleep is disrupted even though they spend a lot of hours in bed.

- Anything that suppresses leptin production or creates resistance to the brain's ability to read leptin signals will make it more difficult for you to control your weight.

The challenge of leptin resistance

If you are getting all the sleep you need, exercise, are watching what you eat and control your calories and still can't lose weight, consider having your leptin levels checked.

Because the amount of leptin circulating is proportional to the amount of fat cells in the body, overweight people have more leptin in their systems than normal weight people do. This can lead to leptin resistance. Basically, despite elevated leptin levels, your brain still doesn't get the message that you're full and satisfied, so your hunger and desire to eat continues.

Leptin resistance isn't well understood yet, but is thought to be very common in people who have a lot of extra fat tissue. If you are in that position and think you could be leptin resistant, the best thing you can do is get advice from a medical professional who works with hormone imbalance. Ask your doctor if you could benefit from seeing an endocrinologist.

High-calorie and sweet foods pose a special danger to the sleep deprived.

When you're tired, it's understandable to reach for a quick pick-me-up, and nothing works like sweet food. Energy drinks and other high-calorie foods lift your energy level, it's true, but they also let you down hard with an energy crash after only 30 to 45 minutes.

What can you do if you are sleep deprived and need to keep going?

- Eat protein. Lean meat, beans and legumes, eggs. Protein will keep you more alert than sugar and you won't have a crash.

- Eat whole grains with high fiber content. Avoid the simple carbohydrates in refined white flour because they metabolize too fast. Whole grains will maintain your energy level longer.

- Plan ahead and have high-protein and whole grain snacks available.

No sleep? Try to avoid the famous See-Food Eat-Food Diet.

For millions of years our ancestors lived with food scarcity. They knew they had to grab whatever food happened to be in front of them. For the thousands of generations who lived without agriculture, being an opportunist meant having the best chance for survival. It also means that we, their descendants, are not bred to resist the food we see. When we see food, we want to eat it. That's how our ancestors survived.

If you haven't slept well, be aware that your self-control is low and your impulse control is weak. Plus, as you now know about your appetite hormones, you'll be feeling hungrier and less satisfied with anything you do eat.

In the United States, fast food, sodas and packaged snacks seem to be selling on every corner and we live surrounded by advertisements to buy them. It's not easy to resist the See-Food Response. How can your commitment to healthy eating survive in this food environment when your resistance is low?

You need tips and techniques to avoid impulsively grabbing whatever food you see in front of you. I've spent years learning how to avoid the See-Food Response, and today feel confident overcoming my cravings and walking away.

Here's my favorite collection of tips that really work for me. They will work for you, too!

	14 TIPS TO HELP YOU AVOID THE SEE-FOOD, EAT-FOOD RESPONSE
Tip #1	Be prepared. Expect that you will have a reaction when you see or smell food. Knowing what to expect helps you manage your response. If you're caught by surprise, it's more difficult to have a practical reaction.
Tip #2	Don't let yourself become overly hungry. Don't skip meals. Prepare to have regular, healthy snacks inbetween meals. Be sure to eat every three hours. Knowing that you've taken care of yourself this way will help you resist reaching for food that you know you really don't need.
Tip #3	Grab a beverage (water, unsweetened tea or coffee, hot water with lemon) as a substitute so your mouth and hands have something to do. If you drink a large glass of water, your stomach will feel full and you'll feel less hungry. This will slow down your rush for food and help you make better choices.
Tip #4	Eat foods high in fiber so they will take longer to digest and you will feel more full longer. Whole fruits and vegetables are a good choice. Remember, fiber only comes from plants.
Tip #5	Eat protein for energy, not sweetened foods and drinks.
Tip #6	Move away from the dessert table! Don't place yourself in the path of temptation. Walk away and distract yourself. Practice saying "No thank you, not today". First say it to yourself. Then, say it out loud when necessary. Saying "no" gets much easier with practice.
Tip #7	If the food is packaged, read both the ingredient and nutrition labels. This will slow you down! Avoid packaged foods if at all possible.
Tip #8	If you're approaching a buffet table or food counter, take at least 60 seconds to look at each and every food available before you reach for anything. Don't start ordering before you've really looked at everything. Take 3 deep breaths and count to 10 before you make your first choice.
Tip #9	Remember portion control! Use a smaller plate, measure your serving very carefully. If it's a dessert, measure by the mouthful, not the plateful. Three mouthfuls maximum!
Tip #10	Do everything possible to avoid seeing high-sugar, high-fat foods so you don't succumb to the see-food, eat-food response. Chew gum if you can't avoid seeing them. Having something already in your mouth will help.

Tip #11	Get at least seven hours of sleep as soon as possible if you are sleep deprived. Count your sleep hours when you wake up. If you have seven hours or more, that's your first success of the day. Celebrate starting the day on a firm, healthy foundation and know that this helps you avoid temptation.
Tip #12	Give yourself positive reinforcement. Remind yourself that when you take care of your other needs successfully, you can also use self-control about food with equal success.
Tip #13	Control as much of your food environment as you can. If you have candy presented in bowls around the office, remove them or ask to have the candy placed in drawers, if possible. If not, pretend the bowls are filled with worms and vomit. Your imagination is powerful. Make it work for you!
Tip #14	Be kind to yourself. It's not easy to get through the day when you're tired. If you impulsively eat something you know is not a good choice for your longterm health, forgive yourself. Learn from what triggered your impulse. Let the experience strengthen your commitment to be more prepared in the future.

YOU ARE NOT ALONE.
OVER 50 MILLION AMERICANS STRUGGLE
TO GET ENOUGH SLEEP.

The Center for Disease Control and Prevention estimates that a staggering 50 to 70 million Americans struggle to get enough sleep every night.

This is a growing public health issue. We all know that driving, flying and running machinery are impaired when the operator is sleep deprived, but it's news to most of us that "Persons experiencing sleep insufficiency are also more likely to suffer from chronic diseases such a hypertension, diabetes, depression and obesity." (Institute of Medicine. *Sleep Disorders and Sleep Deprivation: An Unmet Public Health Problem.* Washington, DC: The National Academies Press; 2006.)

Since this book is focused on helping you control your weight, your need to get enough sleep cannot be overstated. The basic truth is: *lack of sleep will reduce your willpower and increase your appetite.*

If you struggle with impulse control, getting a full night's sleep is an essential management tool.

Here's my own sleep story

I first started being very protective of my sleep when my children were young and I was crazy busy at work. Being torn in two directions—home and work—meant I was always stressed and overcommitted. Most nights I was lucky to sleep five hours. I was completely frazzled. In the evenings I would binge on cookies or ice cream, anything I could find for an energy lift since I was dragging myself through the hours by my fingernails.

Of course my weight was anything but stable. About once a year I would sign up for some kind of diet program and lose 20 to 30 pounds, just enough to make me feel like I was taking care of myself and achieving something important. But the pounds ballooned back on every time I stopped the diet.

I first thought about the benefits of sleep for stress management and gradually became more and more proactive about going to bed on time. I simply needed more sleep to avoid being a short-tempered monster. It wasn't easy to train my family that I must stay in bed for seven hours of sleep, but baring emergencies, they became supportive of me. I'm something of a nightowl, so disciplining myself to go to bed earlier was a major challenge.

Over time, the benefits of being well rested became so obvious in my daily life. I was more clear-headed, made better decisions, had more stamina and self-control. And was so much less stressed. Life still throws me curve-balls (and I've had some doozies) but knowing that my day starts after seven hours of sleep is the foundation I rely on to not be overly rattled and upset.

The first thing I do when I wake up is count my hours of sleep. If it's seven or more, I know I have the reserves to go through the day with willpower and self-control.

I used to overeat in the evenings because I was so tired. When I was able to get consistent sleep, my urge to overeat at night dropped dramatically to manageable levels. And, being prepared with healthy snacks like high-fiber fresh vegetables helps when the munchies strike.

(See *Habit #8: Snack Often* for more information about how to snack and avoid empty calories.)

Getting enough sleep helps me stay focused on my goals and avoid being distracted by temptation.

We live in a hyper-active world, filled with devices that connect us around the clock. Television and websites scream at us to MISS NOTHING. Almost everyone I know, including myself feel that pressure to not be left behind. It's hard to turn off that compulsion to be connected and close our eyes.

By now, I hope I've convinced you that getting enough sleep—seven or more hours a night is an essential habit that will support controlling your weight. Turn off your devices. Tuck yourself in and say goodnight! May all your dreams be sweet dreams!

CAN YOU CATCH UP ON SLEEP? YES! EVEN NAPS WILL IMPROVE YOUR SELF-CONTROL AND REDUCE YOUR APPETITE

The good news is that the damage caused by lack of sleep is reversible! Our brains are incredibly resilient. With just a few nights of solid, uninterrupted sleep, you can:

- Improve how your prefrontal cortex functions and restore its executive ability to set goals and stay on task.

- Restore your will power. Being well rested allows your brain to function at its best. The three prefrontal areas responsible for your willpower work better together and you'll have more self-control if you get at least seven hours of sleep each night.

- Protect yourself from overeating. Sleep helps balance your hormones by decreasing the extra ghrelin released with sleep deprivation.

Getting enough sleep is one of the best things you can do to optimize your willpower and self-control. And there's more good news, If you don't have the lifestyle to support a full-night's sleep, studies have shown that naps can help.

Naps can really help restore your energy

Did you know there's a name for animals that nap instead of sleeping a solid block of hours? "Polyphasic sleepers" is the term and amazingly, 85% of all mammals on Earth sleep this way. We humans are "monophasic sleepers" with our 24 hour days divided clearly into two different periods: awake and asleep.

Some cultures value naps so much that napping in the afternoon is built into the social structure. Think siestas. In the United States, naps are rarely the norm, so when public figures like Presidents John Kennedy and George W. Bush took regular afternoon naps, it was news.

Are nappers just lazy? No. A twenty minute nap can make you more energetic and more productive. If you find yourself sleep deprived at work, do your best to find a private place to lay down your head. You'll have more energy, be in a better mood, be more alert and do a better job.

It's always a good idea to try to catch up on your sleep. And when you're less tired, it's easier to resist eating impulsively.

Get help improving your sleep

Because sleep deprivation is a major issue in American life today, you won't have any trouble finding lots and lots of suggestions on how to make your sleep longer, deeper and more restful. Sleep even has a "Sleep Industry" now, worth $34 billion dollars a year, and growing! Sleep clinics, devices, drugs, books, apps, beds, etc. are all enjoying a growth market.

You can improve your sleep with low cost techniques and not have to spend a lot of money. Many of these techniques require willpower—like going to bed on time or turning off the TV in the bedroom—but we've seen how will power is diminished when you are sleep deprived. This seems like a cruel loop.

If you can, consult a sleep professional. Your doctor is the place to start for help. S/he will determine whether you have a genuine sleep disorder like sleep apnea that needs treatment, or whether you need lifestyle adjustments.

There is no question that getting enough sleep is a challenge. Here are tips and techniques that worked for me to establish consistently getting seven hours of sleep at night.

18 TIPS FOR A BETTER NIGHT'S SLEEP	
Tip #1	Set regular bedtimes and wake up times if you can.
Tip #2	Take time to unwind with bedtime rituals. Be deliberate with your preparations like brushing your teeth and washing your face. Brush your hair with a gentle, relaxing rhythm.
Tip #3	Read in bed for a brief while but avoid bright lights.
Tip #4	Listen to relaxing music if it's on a timer.
Tip #5	Don't exercise strenuously for 3 hours before bedtime. It's important to move your body and get at least 30 minutes of exercise every day, but don't schedule this close to your scheduled sleep time.
Tip #6	Don't start new projects close to bedtime. This will distract and stimulate you, making it harder to settle down for rest.
Tip #7	Cut back on caffeine, especially in the later hours of the day. In addition to coffee, tea and caffeinated sodas, this includes chocolate.
Tip #8	Avoid any form of alcohol before bedtime. No bedtime hot toddies!
Tip #9	Keep your blood sugar balanced. Pay extra attention to avoiding added sugars and simple carbohydrates in the evening. Fiber-rich foods are your best choice.
Tip #10	Control your sleep environment the best you can. Make sure your bed is comfortable and in a sleep-friendly setting. Provide yourself with the best mattress and pillows you can afford. Chose sheets that are comfortable and you enjoy.
Tip #11	Control the lighting where you sleep or wear an eye mask. Blackout curtains are now easily available at Target or other large retailers.
Tip #12	If noise is a problem, consider wearing ear plugs or providing yourself with a white noise device. Ear plugs can take several weeks to get used to, but I personally find them very helpful.
Tip #13	Adjust the temperature in your sleeping room if possible. Being too cold or too hot will interfere with your ability to stay asleep.

Tip #14	Be alert for allergens in your sleep environment. Dust and mold in the air can disturb your rest. Many people are allergic to dust mites. If your nose fills up at night and you have trouble breathing, seek medical attention for help with allergies.
Tip #15	If you have sleep apnea or physical sleep disturbances, seek medical attention. Today's devices like C-Pap machines for apnea sufferers can make a huge positive difference. There's a strong connection between sleep apnea and being overweight, so losing weight is an important way of improving sleep apnea.
Tip #16	Do everything possible to manage daily stress. Breath-focused meditation for at least 5 minutes can calm your mind and relax you. If you're stressed, dedicate 5 minutes of your bedtime preparation time to closing your eyes while breathing deeply. Listening carefully to your breath going in and out. Imagine that your stress is being exhaled with each breath.
Tip #17	If anxieties and concerns are swirling in your mind, keep a notebook handy and write them down before you get into bed. The same holds true for exciting, new ideas.
Tip #18	Have an orgasm at bedtime. Most people find sexual release to be a relaxing, satisfying sleep aid.

HABIT #2
START THE DAY WELL

Eat a breakfast with protein and whole grains
to jump-start your metabolism
What to stock in your kitchen

People who eat breakfast with protein are on average thinner than those who don't eat breakfast, according to the National Weight Control Registry report.

What does this mean for you? If you regularly eat a nutritious breakfast with protein and whole grains you will be more successful controlling your appetite and overeating for the rest of the day.

Why? What happens if you don't eat breakfast? Let's assume that you are lucky to get a full night's sleep, perhaps seven or eight hours. While you are sleeping, your metabolic rate decreases by ten percent. When you skip eating anything in the morning, your body could go perhaps twelve hours without any fuel if lunch is your first food.

Here's where you run into weight-control trouble: If you skip meals, your body senses that it's being starved. You can't control this by thinking—it just happens. Quickly, your metabolism switches into storage mode, and slows the burning of calories to help you through a starvation period.

The best way to keep your metabolism turned on and running is to eat a small nutritious meal first thing in the morning when you wake up.

Skipping breakfast is a terrible idea if you are trying to control your weight.

You may think that you are saving calories by not eating breakfast, but not feeding yourself when you wake up can throw your metabolism off for the entire day. If you want to lose and control your weight at a healthy level, it's time to rethink your morning routines.

There are many reasons why it's easy to be in the habit of skipping breakfast. Perhaps you're in a terrible rush in the morning. Or you might be in the habit of overeating at night then not feeling hungry first thing in the morning. My friend, Anna, eats heavily at night, plus she'll have one or two glasses of wine in the evening. She prefers to go to sleep with her stomach feeling full. It feels comforting to her. But she pays a price for not eating breakfast—after a morning at work she is really hungry at lunchtime and overeats. Anna continues to overeat at dinner and snacks continually throughout the evening. "*I just keep stuffing myself,*" she says. It's a hard cycle to break.

Anna can break the cycle by moving away from heavy food in the evening for just a week and starting to eat a small breakfast. If she plans ahead and prepares something simple to grab in the morning, she'll have less resistance to developing this new habit.

Breakfast doesn't need to be a time-consuming chore. It could be as simple as peanut butter on a rice cake with a glass of milk, or peeling two boiled eggs and eating them with a few whole grain crackers. Or, just reheating your dinner leftovers from the night before. Below, you will find suggestions for quick, nutritious breakfasts that you can eat even on the go.

Avoid eating sugar or sweeteners for breakfast. They will wreck your day.

We are going to discuss sugar more fully in *Habit #6: Avoid Added Sugars and Sweetened Drinks*, but the first place to avoid sugar is the start of your day. Whatever you do, don't reach for that donut! I think of breakfast sweets as toxic and avoid them in all circumstances.

Here's why: Sugar's effect on your body is powerful and after hours of sleeping and not eating, it hits your organs with a bang and sends your metabolism into overdrive. Sugar is actually simple glucose. It quickly floods into your bloodstream, which causes your pancreas to produce insulin to handle the excess. While you're happily remembering that donut, there's an internal battle going on inside your body to balance your blood sugar with insulin spikes. You feel the insulin winning when, an hour after the donut, you feel tired, jumpy and hungry again. Your blood sugar has been tamed to a new, lower level and it's time to eat again.

Do you really need this kind of metabolic drama every morning?

Whole grains, fresh fruit and vegetables are also digested to produce glucose, but when you eat this way, glucose releases into your blood stream more gradually and it's easier for your pancreas to manage. You won't have that quick, wake-me-up sugar spike, but you will feel fuller and better longer. You will be able to manage your appetite and cravings more successfully throughout the day because you didn't wake up your body with a blood sugar battle.

Please don't forget that many products sold as juice have sweeteners, and any fruit juice stripped of natural fiber will be digested just like sugar water. Avoid the juice and eat a piece of whole fruit, instead.

Don't sabotage yourself by starting your day with sugars.

A healthy breakfast helps you start the day with a positive attitude.

There's an added benefit to having a healthy breakfast: you can pat yourself on the back knowing that you've started the day right. It's very encouraging to set your day up for weight control success.

If you start the day with a jelly donut, it's hard to have a positive view of your ability to control yourself. Don't do it! In fact, treating yourself poorly at breakfast can encourage a self-image of being self-destructive. You *know* that donut will not build good health. If you eat it, your poor choice will resonate in your mind for the rest of the day.

Instead, renew your commitment to take good care of your body each morning. Making your first positive choice when you wake up is empowering. For the rest of the day, you know that you can do it!

WHY PROTEIN AND WHOLE GRAINS?
What makes these your best breakfast choices?
It's the Glycemic Index.

Protein and whole grains are low-glycemic index foods. They will take longer to digest and make you feel satisfied longer. This helps you control your appetite.

You have probably heard of the glycemic index (GI), but don't feel badly if you don't fully understand how it works. It's a relatively new system of categorizing food, only proposed for the first time by researchers in the 1980's. Basically, most food that we eat has been assigned a glycemic index number, which describes how fast the food is metabolized and shows up as glucose in blood. ("Blood glucose" is another way of saying "blood sugar".)

A high glycemic index (HGI) means that the food is easy and fast to digest.

A low glycemic number (LGI) means that food takes longer to digest, which is the outcome you want.

Here's why food that digests rapidly is not as good for you: it will elevate your blood glucose quickly and cause your pancreas to make extra insulin. This is called a "spike". Your body will then react to the extra insulin and release hormones to lower the excess supply. Your blood sugar will drop down quickly, or "crash".

When my blood sugar has crashed, I feel uncomfortable, hungry and kind of jumpy. I feel the need to grab something to eat right away. It's much harder for me to make wise choices because I am looking for fast relief from feeling uncomfortable.

The best way I can feel good all morning is to avoid eating sugars. By starting the day with protein and whole grains, I feel comfortable for hours, without hunger, and avoid uncomfortable crashes. Please, give yourself a chance to have a healthy day and start with protein and whole grains.

HOW MUCH PROTEIN DO YOU NEED FOR BREAKFAST?

The amount of protein you need for breakfast should be 25% to 30% of your daily recommended allowance. In my case, it's between 12 and 17 grams of protein, because my daily recommended allowance is 49 grams.

Here's a quick guideline: eat 15 grams of protein with breakfast.

This can be protein from plants (whole cereal grains, beans, nuts, vegetables), or dairy (milk, yogurt, eggs) or animals (chicken, fish, lean red meat—avoid high fat meats). The chart below will list specific foods with grams of protein per portion.

Protein requirements vary with gender, age, activity level. For an average American, The Federal Food and Drug Administration recommends the following for daily protein and calorie intake (RDA):

- Calories: 2,000 calories

- Protein: 50 grams

Calculate your personal calorie and protein recommendations on this website

Averages are useful, but if you want specific recommendations for your age, height, weight and activity levels, there's a very easy online protein calculator:

http://fnic.nal.usda.gov/fnic/interactiveDRI/

This is a free service from the United States Department of Agriculture Food and Nutrition Information Center, which maintains a National Agricultural Library.

It's easy to use, completely anonymous, and will give you nutrition information specifically tailored for your body. In addition to calories and protein recommendations, you will also receive recommendations for fiber and carbohydrate.

Learning how to work these numbers can be confusing, which is why I offered the simple recommendation of 15 grams of protein with breakfast. But, once you accept that getting protein and whole grains for breakfast is critical for weight control, it won't take long to understand how to make this happen.

Here's a screen shot of my own USDA protein calculation:

You Entered:			
Female	Age: 68 yrs	Height: 5 ft. 5 in.	Weight: 135 lbs.
Active		Not Pregnant or Lactating	
Results:			
Body Mass Index (BMI) is 22.5		Estimated Daily Caloric Needs: 2135 kcal/day	

• **About BMI**

Macronutrients

Each reference value refers to *average daily nutrient intake*; day-to-day nutrient intakes may vary.

Macronutrient	Recommended Intake per day
Carbohydrate	240 - 347 grams [1]
Total Fiber	21 grams
Protein	49 grams

HOW TO GET PROTEIN FROM COMMON BREAKFAST FOODS

Protein is measured in grams and milligrams. Learning how to work these numbers can be confusing, which is why I offered the simple recommendation of 15 grams of protein with breakfast. I don't count exact numbers, but rely on a general understanding of which foods are high protein, high fiber and high calorie, then choose my best, most efficient options. (Let's not forget good tasting, too!)

I'm usually moving pretty fast in the morning, and don't have time to fuss with preparing food, so I have a collection of go-to breakfast menus which are included in this chapter.

Here is a quick reference list of everyday breakfast foods and their protein content:

PROTEIN IN COMMON BREAKFAST FOODS
Try to get 15 grams of protein every morning

DAIRY AND DAIRY SUBSTITUTES:

FOOD	PORTION	CALORIES	PROTEIN
Eggs	1 egg	71	6 grams
Cheese (cream)	1 tbsp	49	1 gram
Cheese (cheddar)	1 slice (1 oz)	113	7 grams
Cottage cheese (1% lowfat)	4 oz	81	14 grams
Milk (2% lowfat)	1 cup	86	8 grams
Soy milk	1 cup	132	8 grams
Yogurt (Regular, plain, non-fat)	1 cup	71	6 grams
Yogurt (Greek, plain)	1 cup	100	18 grams

BREADS AND CEREALS (without toppings):

FOOD	PORTION	CALORIES	PROTEIN
Bagel (4 oz, large)	1 bagel	330	12 grams
Bread (choose whole grain)	1 slice	75	3 grams
Cold cereals (whole grain, unsweetened)	1 cup	380	16 grams
English muffin	1 muffin	140	5 grams
Granola (average)	1 cup	598	18 grams
Oatmeal	1 cup	158	6 grams

NUTS, SEEDS AND NUT BUTTERS:

FOOD	PORTION	CALORIES	PROTEIN
Peanut butter	1 tbsp	188	7 grams
Almonds	1 oz	163	6 grams
Sunflower seeds	1 oz	166	5 grams

MEATS AND MEAT SUBSTITUTES*:

FOOD	PORTION	CALORIES	PROTEIN
Bacon	1 slice	46	3 grams
Ham	3 oz	139	14 grams
Sausage (Jimmy Dean Original)	3 links	250	9 grams
Steak	3 oz	158	26
Fish (salmon)	3 oz	103	15 grams
Tofu	3 oz	64	7 grams

*Note that many breakfast meats like bacon and sausage are very fatty and high calorie for the amount of protein they offer. Personally, I avoid them for weight control.

UNUSUAL BREAKFAST CHOICES*:

FOOD (COOKED)	PORTION	CALORIES	PROTEIN
Leftover dinner chicken (no skin or sauce)	2 oz	94	19 grams
Leftover dinner steak	2 oz	105	17 grams
Leftover dinner pork	2 oz	81	15 grams
Beans (average of black, pinto, kidney, lentils, adzuki)	½ cup	114	9 grams
Brown rice	1 cup	216	5 grams

*Note smaller portions of meat than a dinner serving.

Leftovers for breakfast? Why not?

I often eat dinner leftovers for breakfast. They're fast and easy to heat in the microwave, and there's no law that you must eat traditional breakfast foods to start your day. If your dinner was healthy and nutritious, just reheat a smaller portion, and consider putting a handful of green vegetables on your plate for fiber. Reach for a handful of lettuce or kale. It's a great breakfast that's super fast to prepare!

It's important to keep your protein lean.

As much as you love bacon and chicken skin (and I do, too), if you really want to control your weight, you must restrict this kind of fatty material. You don't need to give it up entirely, just hold yourself to one or two small bites. We'll be talking a lot more about controlling how much you eat in *Habit # 3: Learn and Practice Portion Control.*

DON'T FORGET THAT PROTEIN ALSO COMES FROM PLANTS

It seems like the default position in our culture that protein means meat, but vegetarians and vegans can do very well with plant-based proteins. The truth is that your metabolism is very happy with plant-based proteins, which are naturally lean and give you the additional benefit of eating fiber and phytonutrients. (Phytonutrients are micronutrients only present in fruits and vegetables. Some, like carotenoids, act like anti-oxidants.)

All proteins are formed by a combination of amino acids; there are 20 amino acids in what we call a "complete protein". Most meat offers complete proteins, which is what makes eating meat so convenient. Not all plants offer what humans need as complete protein, so if you are a vegetarian or vegan, you know to be careful combining plant food to create a full selection of amino acids. Here's an everyday example of a plant combination which offers complete protein: rice and beans.

There are six plants American shoppers can find fairly easily these days which offer complete or almost complete protein:

- Quinoa: 18 amino acids
- Amaranth: 18 amino acids

- Soybeans: all 20 amino acids
- Buckwheat: all 20 amino acids
- Hempseed: all 20 amino acids
- Chia: 18 amino acids

You will find that these are starting to show up regularly on breakfast cereal shelves, as more people are eating less meat.

Remember: *fiber only comes from plants. There is no dietary fiber in any meat.*

Your goal is 15 grams of protein for breakfast. Add plants (seeds and vegetables) to help you get there.

PROTEIN FROM PLANTS:

FOOD (COOKED)	PORTION	CALORIES	PROTEIN
Amaranth	½ cup	125	5 grams
Bean sprouts	½ cup	24	3 grams
Broccoli	1 cup	98	7 grams
Buckwheat	½ cup	293	12 grams
Chia seeds	1 oz	137	4 grams
Edamame	1 cup	240	17 grams
Hempseed	1 tbsp	40	5 grams
Kale	1 cup	34	3 grams
Lentils	1 cup	230	18 grams
Oats	1 cup	158	6 grams
Peas (green)	1 cup	117	9 grams
Peppers (red or green)	1 medium	30	2 grams
Potato	1 medium	110	4 grams
Quinoa	½ cup	148	5 grams
Spinach	1 cup	7	3 grams
Soy beans (complete protein)	1 cup	298	29 grams

Potatoes are common for breakfast
but watch out for added fats

We love our hash browns and home fries. People rarely eat a dry potato for breakfast, which is why I make the yummy home fries a treat, not a daily dish. There are 110 calories in a medium dry potato but only 3 grams of protein and 2 grams of fiber. Each tablespoon of butter will add 100 calories. Fry your potatoes in oil, and you'll add 150 calories per tablespoon. That's a lot of calories for 3 grams of protein. (In Habit #5: *Know What's in the Food You Eat* we'll discuss what to know about calories.)

What about fruits? Yes, we love fruit for breakfast!

I eat fruit almost every morning with breakfast, but the protein content is negligible. Fresh fruit is delicious, offers vitamins, minerals, phytonutrients and fiber. There are many health benefits to eating fruit, and most nutritionists recommend 2 to 3 cups of fruit every day.

I do not recommend eating a breakfast of just fruit. Your body will digest it faster than protein and whole grains. Eat fruit *with* your breakfast but don't eat fruit *for* your breakfast. Don't let fruit be the substitute for the protein you need to start your day right.

Suggestions for eating fresh and dried fruit will be covered in *Habit #8: Snack Often.*

BREAKFAST FOODS TO AVOID
If you want to lose pounds and control your weight,
don't eat sugars for breakfast!

If you want to lose and control your weight, do not eat sweetened foods in the morning. Do not eat sweet packaged cereals no matter what the box says. Read every label like your life depends on it. Seek out whole foods, not packaged foods.

But….what about beautiful breakfast pastries? Croissants? Bear claws? Cinnamon rolls? Coffee cakes? I love them, I do. It's really hard to say "no". Having a breakfast pastry as an occasional treat is fine, especially if you cut it in half and only eat half. It's hard to give these up! But, absolutely, positively, do not eat breakfast pastries every day.

Sugars and refined white flours will not give you the nutrition you need to be healthy and control your weight. We will discuss both in the following chapters, *Habit #6: Avoid Added Sugars and Sweetened Drinks*, and *Habit #7: Find Substitutes for Refined White Flour*.

AVOID EATING THESE FOR BREAKFAST:

FOOD	PORTION	CALORIES	PROTEIN
Cereal (boxed, ready to eat, sweetened)	1 cup	144	2 grams
Donuts (of any kind)	1 glazed donut	360	2 grams
Danish pastry or any sweetened pastry	1 medium	262	4 grams
Muffins	1 medium	426	5 grams
Pancakes/waffles with syrup, and butter	2	520	8 grams
Elaborate sweetened coffees (Ex: Starbucks Mocha Frappuccino®)	16 oz	410	5 grams

LEARN TO LOVE WHOLE GRAINS
Whole grain is not the same as whole wheat or multi-grain

Food producers don't make it easy. Bread labels are especially confusing with descriptions about "whole wheat" or "whole wheat flour". If you want to eat whole grain foods, you need to find the words "whole grain" in the ingredients. Don't be tricked by brown colored bread, since food processors can color the bread with molasses.

What exactly is a whole grain?

Whole grain is the entire seed of a grain plant (wheat, oat, barley, rice, millet, etc.) that has all of its original parts in the same proportions that it had in nature. It may be ground up into flour but nothing has been removed by processing.

The seed contains three basic parts and all must be present in whole grain products:

- **Bran:** The outside layer of the kernel.

- **Endosperm:** The largest part of the kernel, inside the bran.

- **Germ:** The fertile, reproductive part of the kernel.

The bran and germ are the most important, nutritious part of the seed. They are rich in protein and fiber and also contains vitamins such as Vitamin E, folic acid, B vitamins (Niacin, Thiamin and B6) and minerals (including iron, magnesium, selenium and zinc).

In contrast, the endosperm is mostly starch, simple carbohydrates and contains little in the way of other nutrients. When you eat flour made from ground endosperm (all refined flours) you get very little besides calories.

Refined white flour contains only the endosperm

Refined white flour has been stripped of the grain's most valuable parts—the bran and germ with all their fiber and proteins have been removed. This process creates flour that is easy to work with and is pleasant pale color, which is especially useful for cakes and pastries. As our food supply became more industrialized, creating flour that was standardized really helped bakers make more products for less money. But, while this is fine for the producers' profit margin, it left the buying public with baked food stripped of vital nutrients. That's why you see the word "Fortified" on many bread labels. Producers are adding vitamins and minerals back into the blanched, stripped flour.

Wouldn't it be better to eat the food as nature intended? Personally, I don't trust chemists to give me a full range of vitamins, minerals and micronutrients. I trust Mother Nature!

Make the effort to find bread that says "whole grain" on the label.

For optimal weight control, avoid white bread, in its many forms. This is especially hard in restaurants where most toast and breadbaskets are basically refined white flour. And then there's hamburger buns and pizza crusts. Even ordering a sandwich can be a challenge, which is why I usually choose a wrap instead of bread slices. For breakfast out, if you eat pancakes or waffles, expect to be served white flour.

While wheat dominates our bread production, Americans rarely eat wheat as a loose grain the same way we eat rice. Bread is very convenient for us. It's available everywhere, has predictable tastes and there's a bread for every budget.

Think beyond toast! When you eat oatmeal for breakfast, you have already expanded your menu beyond wheat. Consider trying hot cereals with other grains such as amaranth, buckwheat and barley as well. Much of the world's population starts the day with rice. For me, whole grain rice cakes are very useful for breakfast.

The benefits of whole grain

Why are whole grains so important? To be healthy, our bodies require fiber, vitamins, minerals, proteins and enough calories to stay strong. Whole grains contain all of these. The fiber is especially important. It slows down your digestion so your blood sugar stays steady, longer. And, we all know that eating fiber helps material move through our colon and bowels to keep us regular.

And, sodium is so low in whole grains that the USDA only catches it as a trace element. For those of you advised to eat a low sodium diet, whole grains are a good choice.

Whole grains are versatile food that belongs in every kitchen and on every menu. They are easy to cook, keep in your cabinet without refrigeration when they're dry, combine very well with vegetables, meats and sauces and…the best part…they are delicious.

Here is a list of 14 whole grains which are becoming more familiar to food buyers and cooks. I've only included one variety of wheat, although if you look around, there are many varieties available.

TRY THESE WHOLE GRAINS
They are rich in fiber, protein, vitamins and minerals

NUTRIENTS IN WHOLE GRAINS*:

WHOLE GRAIN (Cooked)	PORTION	CALORIES	PROTEIN	FIBER	VITAMINS & MINERALS
Amaranth	¾ cup	167	6.1 grams	3.0 grams	Iron, Calcium, Selenium, Magnesium, Phosphorus, Vit C, B3, B5, B6
Buckwheat	¾ cup	154	5.9 grams	4.5 grams	Magnesium, Potassium, Phosphorus, B2, B3
Barley (hulled)	¾ cup	159	5.6 grams	7.8 grams	Potassium, Copper, Phosphorus, Manganese, Selenium, B1, B3
Cornmeal	¾ cup	163	3.6 grams	3.3 grams	Iron, Magnesium, Phosphorus, Manganese, Selenium, B1, B3, B5
Millet	¾ cup	170	4.9 grams	5.7 grams	Magnesium, Phosphorus, Copper, Manganese, B1, B3
Oats	¾ cup	171	5.9 grams	4.5 grams	Iron, Magnesium, Phosphorus, Zinc, Copper, Manganese, Selenium, B1, B3, B5, Folate B9
Rice (brown)	¾ cup	166	3.5 grams	1.6 grams	Magnesium, Phosphorus, Manganese, Selenium, B1, B3, B6

Rice (wild)	¾ cup	161	6.6 grams	2.8 grams	Manganese, Phosphorus, B5, B6, Folate B9
Rye	¾ cup	152	4.6 grams	6.8 grams	Iron. Phosphorus, Potassium, Manganese, Zinc, B3
Sorghum	¾ cup	162	3.5 grams	3.0 grams	Iron, Magnesium, Potassium, Selenium, B3, B5
Spelt (Farro grande)	¾ cup	152	6.5 grams	4.8 grams	Iron, Phosphorus, Potassium, Zinc, Copper, Manganese, Thiamin, B3
Quinoa	¾ cup	166	6.3 grams	3.2 grams	Iron, Magnesium, Phosphorus, Zinc, Manganese, B1, B3, B6, Folate B9
Wheat (durum)	¾ cup	153	6.1 grams	4.8 grams	Iron, Magnesium, Phosphorus, Potassium, Zinc, Manganese, Selenium, B1, Be, B6

*All data comes from the USDA Nutrient Database. ¾ Cup of cooked whole grains is equal to 45 grams of dry grains. It is assumed that all grains have been cooked in water. All grains listed have many more vitamins and minerals, but only the ones present in the largest quantities have been listed.

Even with our long history with grains, there is still so much to learn

Agriculture started thousands of years ago with cereal grain crops. Humans cultivated grain (wheat, barley, rice, maize) before we learned to grow anything else, so we've had longer to study and learn about grains than any other crops. Historically, growing grain allowed our ancestors to settle down in cities and thrive. Extra supplies of grain gave city dwellers the freedoms to develop specialized labors, such as writing, and created wealth through trading with other cities.

It was grain that developed the first alcohol for people to drink. Beer is thought to have been fermented from grain 12,000 years ago!

But despite our very long history with grains, figuring out the relationships between the human body and the foods we eat remains a complex challenge. Consider that vitamins weren't even discovered until the 1930's. My mother and father were both born before anyone knew that Vitamins A, B, C or D even existed.

Understanding nutrition has become so important because, as American consumers, we are now presented with a bewildering variety of food and "food" choices. In our daily eating, fast foods and processed foods have replaced whole, nutritionally rich foods like whole grains. Every supermarket is filled with "vitamin enriched" or "protein enriched" packaged foods. Even water is now sold to us with added vitamins.

But taking a vitamin here and a protein there and putting them together in a processed material is just not as complete as eating whole foods as nature intended. Who would you rather trust—a chemist with limited knowledge or Mother Nature?

Eating whole grains, either cooked intact or ground into flour, is eating the best that Nature can give us, especially if you eat organic. Don't allow yourself to be cheated out of the bran and the germ. Demand your full portion of grain nutrients. Ask your grocer for more whole grain products. Choose the whole grain option at restaurants when you see it. Even fast food vendors can be influenced because suppliers are very sensitive to market demand. When more customers demand a variety of whole grains, suppliers will respond.

Remember, don't be fooled by words on the label. It must say "whole grain" not just "whole wheat".

A word about gluten

Wheat contains gluten, which many people are trying to avoid eating. If you suffer from Celiac Disease or are just cutting back on gluten, you probably already know about other whole grains including amaranth, millet, oats, sorghum or quinoa and have them in the house. All whole grain choices are a fine way to start your day.

My friend, Natalie, has Celiac Disease so she avoids wheat and makes the effort to keep other grains pre-cooked in her refrigerator. "*I usually start the day with organic pure oatmeal which is quick and easy to fix in the microwave and great with fruit and plain yogurt on the top. If I'm in a real rush, peanut butter on a rice cake is my best friend.*"

My understanding about why many people who do not have Celiac Disease but are sensitive to wheat is this: hybridized wheat is a modern creation and contains proteins not present in ancient grains. Some people are sensitive and react poorly to those proteins. There are also new strains of yeast used to process wheat, which result in new compounds in the final product.

I am severely allergic to many tree nuts including walnuts, which could kill me if I ate them. It's the proteins in the nuts that my body reacts to. So, based on my own experience, I can easily believe that some people shouldn't eat gluten and wheat of any kind. That said, there are many other people who have not researched the matter thoroughly and have just hopped on "gluten-free" as a fad.

In the community of people I know, there are both types of gluten-free eaters: those with Celiac or genuine sensitivities, and those who hop on one diet fad after another. As always, my very strong advice is to do your homework! Research and understand what you're eating and chose carefully.

And, I applaud how the demand for gluten-free products has made other fine grains like spelt and millet much more readily available. Another positive result is that more people have become aware of our industrialized food chain and the dangers of processed foods. Hopefully, this will result in increased demand for organic, whole food.

HERE'S WHAT IS ALWAYS STOCKED IN MY KITCHEN FOR BREAKFAST

Keeping these 14 foods in your kitchen is not just about providing you with healthy breakfast choices, it's about giving you freedom to relax in the morning knowing that you have what you need.

Every single one of these foods has a long shelf life. Nothing is going to spoil in two or three days. You can buy these to stock your kitchen once a week, or even once every other week.

Keep these breakfast foods in your cabinet and refrigerator and you will always be ready to start the day right:

BREAKFAST FOOD	QUANTITY	COMMENT
Whole grain cereal (cold)	1-2 boxes	Read the label carefully. Watch out for high-calorie granolas.
Whole grain cereal (hot)	1-2 boxes	Cook with water, chopped apple and top with Greek yogurt for a delicious breakfast. I add "pumpkin pie" spices for added taste. Find good varieties of whole grain cereals at Trader Joe's.
Milk, soy milk or almond milk	1 container	Watch out for sweeteners in soy milk.
Eggs	1 doz	Buy organic if you can.
Eggs (hard boiled)	1 doz	Prepare boiled eggs for a super-quick grab-and-go breakfast.
Butter or butter substitute	1 lb	I use a yogurt-based substitute but also stock butter for cooking great tasting omelets for guests.
Salt and pepper	Shaker & grinder	Easiest way to season eggs.
Yogurt	1 container	Plain, whole milk Greek Yogurt is my favorite and has a higher protein content than non-Greek yogurts. Avoid yogurts with added fruits and sugar. Add your own jam or chopped fresh fruit. Whole milk yogurts are rich and so much better tasting than 2% or non-fat.

Fruit (apples, oranges, melon)	Several	Keep a fruit bowl on your kitchen counter. Apples are especially useful in the morning to add to cereals, or cut and take slices with you for a mid-morning snack. We always have apples and oranges in our kitchen. Melons are a special weekend treat.
Peanut butter or almond butter	1 jar	Unsweetened. Make sure there are no added sweeteners. Read the label!
Jam, preserves or fruit spread	1 jar	Use sparingly. Spread very thin over peanut butter or toast. Find whole fruit preserves and avoid high-sugar jellies.
Whole grain bread	1 loaf	Experiment until you find one that you really like. If whole grain is hard to find in your supermarket, talk to the manager. Bread freezes well so if you have room in your freezer you can stock an extra loaf.
Whole grain rice cake	1 container	Very useful as a substitute for toast, and will keep longer in your cabinet.
Protein powder	1 container	Add to milk (or milk substitute) for super-quick breakfast drink. Add to vegetable or fruit smoothies. Vanilla is most neutral flavor but to drink protein powder on its own, I prefer chocolate.

BREAKFAST BEVERAGES AND WEIGHT CONTROL

Here are some specific recommendations for breakfast beverages to optimize your weight control lifestyle.

Drink a glass of water first thing in the morning, and have more energy

While you're sleeping, your body uses water so you wake up naturally dehydrated. If you drink a glass of water first thing in the morning, you will rehydrate and boost your energy levels.

It's an easy routine to establish. Just leave an 8 oz glass next to your sink and have a glass of water before you brush your teeth. Whether the water is warm or cold doesn't matter. Personally, I prefer warm water because it's easier on my stomach.

Over the years, there have been many claims that drinking water has nearly miraculous results. It will flush out toxins, increase the elasticity of your skin and drinking ice water will help you burn more calories. Who knows. I haven't seen any credible proof. But, I do know that drinking a glass of fresh water on an empty stomach helps me get ready for the day. And….it is certain….more water in your system definitely helps with constipation.

Coffee or tea? Yes, please!

If you're like me, morning doesn't really start without coffee. Morning coffee is a requirement at my house and a considerable amount of kitchen counter space is dedicated to preparing it. Or, if I'm out, finding the nearest coffee house for a strong morning cup is a top priority!

The weight control key is learning to drink coffee unsweetened. I use milk or soy milk and no sweetener of any kind, thanks to months of practicing drinking my coffee that way. This may seem like a lot of effort, but consider that over a year you will save thousands of calories, especially if you drink more than one cup each day.

I recommend learning to give up artificial sweeteners, too. Splenda, Equal, Sweet 'N Lo just maintain your appetite for sweetened foods. You can learn to overcome wanting sweeteners with practice, with the added benefit of reducing your consumption of additives and chemicals.

Learning to give up sweetener in coffee wasn't an easy change for me, but now unsweetened coffee seems perfectly natural. And desirable. When I'm at Starbucks or Peet's, I'll order an Americano (espresso with hot water) to avoid sweetened drinks, which no longer appeal either for taste or health. They are like drinking dessert.

Sweeteners in your coffee are hard to avoid—temptations are everywhere you go. All restaurants will offer sweeteners to you in one form or another. Yesterday, I was at lunch and when coffee was served, cubes of sugar were already on the cup's saucer.

If you use non-diary creamers like Coffee-Mate in powdered or liquid form, just know that they contain a lot of sugar or high fructose products.

The theme that *you can learn to love different tastes* will be covered repeatedly in this book. Learning to love coffee without sugar was a big shift for me but I have no regrets. Have patience and keep trying. You can do it, too!

Juice: Sold as healthy but the reality is more complex

You wouldn't drink sugar water for breakfast, but that's what many juice and juice-like products come down to. As always, read the label and never buy a "juice" that has added sweeteners.

Most juice contains no pulp or fiber, and hits your system fast, jerks up your blood sugar, which results in an insulin spike as your body struggles bringing your blood sugar levels back to acceptable levels. Pulp is fiber which slows digestion. In addition to keeping your blood sugar levels more stable, fiber allows your digestive system to do a better job of extracting nutrients as the fiber-slowed material moves through your gut.

So, if possible, do not buy and drink juices without pulp. Drink unfiltered apple juice or orange juice with a lot of pulp. If you can see right through the bottle, that juice has no pulp. Avoid pretty colored, transparent juices.

Eating a whole piece of fruit is always a better weight control choice than drinking juice. Keep in mind that some whole fruit, such as pineapple and mango, are naturally very high in sugar.

Make your own juice

Many books are available about the benefits of juicing, and I believe that juice freshly made has to be better than older juice out of containers, since vitamins and enzymes in juice are subject to oxidation and deterioration. And anyone who has tasted fresh-squeezed orange juice certainly knows that the taste is so much more delicious.

It's a big advantage to be able to create your own blend of juices. (Apple-celery-carrot is my personal favorite.) Note that different fruits and vegetables required different types of juicers. Apples and oranges aren't passed through the same piece of equipment, so if you do decide to get a juicer, consider which fruits and vegetables you prefer and do research on the best brand to juice them.

There are many types of electric juicers available, but reading their reviews recently, I was struck by how a common goal is to maximize the juice yield while minimizing pulp. This is not a good weight control idea! Pulp is fiber and you want to eat fiber, especially in the morning. Fiber in your breakfast will help you feel full and satisfied longer.

For this reason, for those of you who wish to drink your fruit with breakfast, I recommend smoothies.

Smoothies: Why they are a better breakfast choice than juice

The primary difference between juice and smoothies is that smoothies are made in a blender with the whole fruit or vegetable. All parts, juice and pulp, are blended together so you get the full benefit of eating whole foods. (Although you do have to core the apples and pull out pits from stone fruit.)

The easiest way to have fruit always ready for breakfast smoothies is to buy large bags of frozen berries. They'll keep in your freezer and are ready for you to pour a cupful in the blender. Add a fresh apple or banana and you have a wonderful blend of whole fruits.

Add protein powder and you can drink your breakfast. A scoop of plain yogurt adds creaminess. All of this goodness takes just minutes to prepare.

Another advantage of smoothies is that the equipment required—a blender—is useful in the kitchen for other food preparation. If you don't have a blender now, consider buying one. We use a Blendtec TB-621-20, with a strong 1,560 watt motor. Vitamix is another popular powerful blender. On Amazon, you can find a wide range of brands, priced from $29.99 to over $600. Read the reviews and buy the highest watt motor you can afford.

Children delight in helping to prepare morning smoothies, which makes smoothies a good family choice. Just remember to hold back the sweeteners. You can even get them to drink their spinach if you blend it with fruit!

My friend, Robert, who has a busy job in computer science with a long commute, keeps a $79 NutriBullet personal blender on his kitchen counter. In his morning rush, he throws a banana, a handful of frozen blueberries, a cup of milk and a scoop of protein powder into the top of his NutriBullet, which converts to a travel cup that he grabs on his way out the door.

Where smoothies run into weight control trouble is when sweeteners and sweet frozen yogurts are added. It's tempting to add sweeteners but do your best to retrain your taste preferences and avoid the sweeteners. Often, protein powders already include sweeteners—they are very hard to avoid in those products. Read the label and do the best you can. If your protein powder has sweeteners, use it but don't add any more sugar, honey or syrup.

BREAKFAST BARS? ARE THEY A GOOD CHOICE?

Packaged breakfast bars are packaged foods which means you must read the label carefully. The breakfast bars at your supermarket breakfast section are unlikely to be whole grain and probably contain added sugar, fats and salt.

I never buy breakfast bars in the breakfast section.

A better choice are the high-protein energy bars, sold with the snack foods. They often average 300 calories with up to 20 grams of protein. Some have a high fiber count. The downside is that most taste like candy bars and have a lot of carbohydrates.

Nevertheless, I always have a few energy bars in my snack drawer to grab for breakfast if I'm really in a time emergency. I often keep one in my car, if there's a long drive coming up. And, if I'm out and need a snack mid-morning or mid-afternoon, you can almost always find a reliable brand of energy bar at gas station stores and newsstands. This will always be a better choice than a bag of chips or a candy bar!

Packaged foods are always the last choice if whole foods are available, but sometimes you're stuck and need to make compromises. I travel a lot and often find myself in unknown places without access to the foods I prefer. Planning ahead and carrying food with you helps, but that's not always possible. Energy bars can be a useful substitute.

BUSINESS TRAVEL: WHAT TO HAVE FOR BREAKFAST?

Protein powder is a great choice when you're on the road

If your work requires frequent travel, you are at the mercy of hotel breakfasts. This may work out well if you can order eggs (no fatty bacon, please) and dry toast (this won't be whole grain). Many business hotels/motels offer a continental breakfast which is usually dominated by refined white flour and sugar. Eating this stuff is dangerous for you. I appreciate that it's "free food", included in the price of the room so it's doubly tempting.

Sometimes, the continental breakfast includes hard-boiled eggs and fruit. Grab two eggs and an apple. Keep the sweeteners out of your coffee. Eat a plain yogurt in the little plastic cup. You're good to go.

Avoid looking at the other guests with the gooey Danish, oily muffin or syrupy waffle on their plates.

I recommend buying a high quality protein powder and traveling with it, even if your trip is only an overnight. You can carry your daily portions easily in a zipped plastic bag. And, you can avoid being tempted by sweet morning pastries that will taste great for a minute, but will sabotage your long-term efforts.

For my entire career, I travelled frequently on business, staying in wide range of places, from the lowest budget motels to elegant five star hotels. Admittedly, it's hard to walk away from an opulent breakfast at a five star hotel, and I usually didn't. You're safe if you stick to eggs, vegetables, fruit or oatmeal, and avoid added sugars and the yummy pastries. And…if you order an omelet, go light on the cheese!

For most business trips I brought my own 8 ounce plastic glass, and a spoon to stir my protein powder. Avoiding the average hotel breakfast was a big relief and better for my weight control campaign than depending on my will power after walking into the breakfast room. I avoided temptation entirely! And when I stepped out of the hotel door, it was great knowing that I had taken good care of myself.

Buy protein powder at GNC, Trader Joe's, Costco, Whole Foods or any health food store. You can even order it on Amazon. Read the ingredients carefully for added sweeteners.

BE WILLING TO TRY SOMETHING NEW. YOUR TASTE CAN BE RETRAINED IF YOU KEEP TRYING.

You can expect to not like the flavor of your new food choices if you have been used to a diet that is sweet, salty and full of fat.

Virtually the only flavor that humans like instantly is a sweet taste. Personally, I love sweet foods, but I love my size 8 hips more and I know that sweets and fats must be limited. It's not easy to retrain your tastes as an adult so you deserve praise for being willing to try!

Making adjustments is a basic part of changing your lifestyle from one that promotes being overweight to one that incorporates habits that will control your weight. Learning to eat foods that are not full of sugar and fat is a basic part of this change. It will be easier for you if you're realistic: it won't be easy. Some people have food addictions and need professional help. Others just need practice, lots of practice.

Let's take a look at yogurt, a food that most people think is healthy and good for you. Please don't give up on plain yogurt as your best choice. If you are used to eating yogurt with sugary fruit added, it's like eating a sweet dessert. It may take you a while to adjust to the taste of plain yogurt because a typical 6 ounce yogurt container has 20 grams of sugar. (This might be listed on the ingredients as "evaporated cane juice".)

In *Part One: Start by Learning Why You are Unique*, we discussed taste preferences, how learning to like new foods takes multiple tastings. The magic number is fifteen. Don't give up on plain yogurt until you have sincerely tried it at least fifteen times. You'll be surprised—it will start tasting reasonable and normal to you.

Just remember, you <u>will</u> adjust to new flavors. Transition times don't last forever.

HABIT #3
EXERCISE FOR 30 MINUTES EVERY DAY.

Teach yourself that a day without
exercise is a day that's incomplete
Learn to fidget

You've heard by now that exercise is like the magic cure for so many modern ailments. For those of us who struggle with weight control, exercise is an essential part of our day. <u>It's not optional</u>, especially if you spend most of your time sitting down.

Exercise doesn't need to be fancy or stressful—you can start at a level that's comfortable for you. Basically, all you need to start a regular exercise program is moving your body for thirty minutes a day. Everyday? Yes, to control your weight, you need to move an average of thirty minutes every day.

The Center for Disease Control says that walking for ten minutes three times a day will satisfy the daily goal. All you need to do is find three spaces of ten minutes to start moving every day!

My very strong recommendation is that you don't try to game the system by adding minutes from one day onto the next. If you can exercise 45 minutes on Monday, don't pull 15 minutes from Tuesday. Just congratulate yourself that you exceeded your Monday goal.

I've seen friends outsmart themselves counting minutes and trying to justify how a two hours of exercise will last all week. It won't. Anyone who wants to learn more about the physiology of exercising should definitely do research. For the rest of us, just accepting that we need to move our bodies at least thirty minutes every day is a good way to built a life-style dedicated to weight control.

Of course, you should check with your doctor before starting any new exercise program.

Are you embarrassed about how you look? Does shame hold you back from exercising?

I've heard that one in four women were nervous and reluctant to exercise in public because they feel badly about how they look.

Let's overcome embarrassment! Don't let yourself be shamed! Refuse to allow worry about other people's judgments overpower your need to care for your body. *Your needs are more important than imagining what other people think.* They may not even be paying attention to you—most people are too busy thinking about themselves. That's exactly what you need to do: think about yourself and your need to control your weight. Don't let shame hold you back.

Why is thirty minutes every day an exercise minimum?

The effect of exercise on the body is the subject of centuries of study and is still not fully understood except that it's healthy for many reasons. We're going to cover just a few of the benefits, because this book is about general weight control solutions, not about highly detailed exercise analysis.

If you are resisting the need for daily exercise and want to deny or argue about the benefits, consider that you may be willfully obstructing your path to weight control. Accepting the need to do something you really don't want to do is a major challenge, but those of us who know that we have to make adjustments in our lives in order to control our weight, just move ahead anyway.

It's OK to hate exercising. It's not OK to avoid doing it. Just do it.

Kaiser Permanente, often ranked as the premier integrated health care provider in the United States, recommends 150 minutes of exercise per week. That's two and a half hours per week. I'm a member of Kaiser, and every doctor or health care provider I see there asks: "Are you exercising 150 minutes a week? And if not, how many minutes?" Since I exercise a minimum of 30 minutes every day, that's a total of 210 minutes each week. Minimum. More is better, I think.

Keeping a running weekly tally works for some people but not me. It's easier for me to think about exercise on a daily basis. I just accept that I need to exercise no less than thirty minutes every day. That way, even if I miss a day, my minutes still far above Kaiser's recommended exercise totals.

FIVE TOP REASONS WHY REGULAR EXCERISE MATTERS FOR WEIGHT CONTROL

Let's focus on specific benefits that regular exercise will give you for weight control.

Reason #1: Exercise burns calories:

When you move your body, it takes energy in the form of calories. The more you move, the more calories you will burn.

When you eat, you put calories into your body. So, it's simple addition and subtraction: If you burn more than you eat, you will lose weight. If you eat more than you burn, you will gain weight. If you burn more, you can eat more, if that's your choice.

Reason #2: Exercise strengthens and builds your muscles:

Muscles are the most metabolically active part of your body and, pound for pound, will burn more calories than organs. It's challenging to think about the inside of our bodies, underneath our skin. There's so much focus on organs, like our hearts, our brains, our kidneys, that unless you're an athlete, you may not have learned about the metabolic role of your muscles.

Your muscles demand energy to keep moving. Most of your organs are just going along for the ride. The more you use your muscles, the more calories you will burn. That's why most personal trainers focus on strength-building exercises with weights to help your muscles reach their peak performance.

An added benefit is that once your muscles are warmed up, they keep demanding energy and will continue to use more calories.

Your muscles are your best friends and allies for weight control, especially the large muscle groups in your legs and abdomen. The more you learn to keep them moving, the easier it will be to control your weight.

Reason #3: Exercise changes your metabolism in a good way. It protects your heart and brain and improves your mood.

It's no secret that exercise is recommended to help control high blood pressure and cholesterol. Here's why: Being active increases your body's production of high-density lipoprotein (HDL), the "good" cholesterol. It also decreases your unhealthy triglycerides.

Moving matters to your body. If you have consulted with a doctor about heart disease, diabetes, metabolic syndrome, arthritis and a variety of other health issues, you have certainly been told that exercise is an important part of building your health.

Exercise also changes the chemistry in your brain in a good way. Feeling blue? Depressed? Frustrated with the challenges in your life? Go for a brisk 30 minute walk. Moving your legs will increase your heart rate and pump more oxygen to your brain. Increased activity also releases hormones that have anti-depression effects.

One of my neighbors, Alice, is raising a son with autism. It's been very stressful and challenging. Alice has told me that if it weren't for being able to exercise vigorously for an hour a day, she would have been too stressed and depressed to function effectively. *"Being able to swim a mile is what kept my sanity,"* she said. *"I came out of the pool exhausted, but with my spirit refreshed and optimistic. It was like magic. On days without my own exercise, I could feel my spirits sinking lower and lower. But, after I swam a mile, I felt self-confident and knew I could handle anything."*

Reason #4: Want better sex? Move your body more during the day!

There are so many reasons that moving your body will improve your sex life, with a partner or whether you are pleasuring yourself.

Studies have shown that women become aroused more easily and deeply if they have regular exercise. Don't you want more and better orgasms? Well, get off the couch and go walk for thirty minutes every day!

Exercise improves your circulation, makes your arms and legs more flexible, improves your stamina, and gives your confidence moving your body.

While you exercise, you can also be thinking kind thoughts about yourself. Think encouraging thoughts that your body is a source of pleasure, and know that the more you exercise, the better you will look and feel.

Reason #5: You will sleep better if you exercise daily.

Moving your body for at least thirty minutes affects your internal body temperature. Exercise will raise your body temperature which then will boomerang back down even lower than if you hadn't exercised at all. Scientists think that it's the lower body temperature that helps you sleep more deeply.

To get the best sleep benefit, exercise in the late afternoon or early evening, assuming that you sleep at night. Avoid exercising in the three hours before you go to bed because your heart, brain and muscles will be too stimulated to settle down quickly.

Better sleep has many benefits that are discussed further in *Habit #1: Get Enough Sleep.*

Walking is the easiest way to start

Walking is free. You don't need to sign up for a gym membership or buy a special outfit. You need sturdy, good-fitting shoes, of course. Also sunscreen for your face and a jacket for chilly days. That's it.

You may think that the tricky part is finding the time, but the real challenge is finding the will to start moving.

My friend, Colleen, lives in Manhattan. She used to take the subway to work. Now, she gets up 30 minutes earlier in the morning and walks 3 miles to work every day, rain or shine. Colleen has struggled with her weight and for years has hovered around 200 pounds. Over the course of a year, walking to work Monday through Friday, and not eating sugar (we'll get to that), she lost over 50 pounds and has kept it off for 5 years. She is at her Weight Watcher's goal weight for the first time in 20 years!

LEARN TO FIDGET: ADD MOVEMENT TO YOUR DAY

Let's consider what you can do if you have a long commute or are required to sit for many hours. How can you keep your body moving? The answer is learn to fidget.

Don't consider exercise as an isolated event in your day. The more you keep your body moving—at any level of intensity—the easier it will be for you to control your weight. All movement burns calories. The more you move your muscles during the day, the more energy your body is forced to provide and the more calories you will burn.

Studies consistently show that people who fidget are thinner.

You can flex your butt muscles or wiggle your feet without anyone noticing. Well, if your butt muscles are very developed, you will raise yourself two inches higher in your chair, so your coworkers might notice. If you're in a car, on a bus or subway, nobody will see a thing. I do butt flexes regularly whenever I'm sitting at my desk, and while I'm driving, waiting for a stop light. After so many years of butt flexes, seeing a stop light is almost an automatic trigger!

If you don't mind more movement, jiggle in your seat. Shake your shoulders and wiggle your fanny. If you want total secrecy, tense your stomach muscles, flex your thighs or do vaginal kegels. There's a fidget for every circumstance, whether you're standing, sitting or laying down.

Fidgeting is not a substitute for regular exercise but learning to fidget at every available opportunity will help tone your muscles and even make exercise easier.

NINE FAVORITE WAYS TO FIDGET

You can fidget with most muscles in your body. From wiggling your feet to shrugging your shoulders, fidgeting can be done anywhere. There are even fidgets you can do so no one will notice, like tensing your calf muscles.

Fidget #1: Work your butt:

Sit up straight in your chair with both feet on the floor. Make sure that your feet are lined up evenly. Tense both sides of your butt at once, as hard as you can. You will feel the squeeze moving down the top of your thigh. As you get stronger, your squeezes will have more power and you will feel yourself lifting from your seat. You are working your gastrocnemius muscle.

Squeeze both side five times. Now alternate, first squeeze your right butt and then squeeze your left butt. Do this five times.

Repeat often throughout the day.

Learn more: The butt has three gluteal muscles: the gluteus maximus, gluteus medius and gluteus minimus. This kind of butt squeeze works the gluteus maximus and will help tone and tighten your butt.

Fidget #2: Flex your thighs:

Sit up straight in your chair with both feet on the floor. Tense the top of your right thigh. You will find that it's hard to do without also tensing the bottom of your thigh. Practice isolating the muscles on top and squeezing them as hard as you can. Switch to the left leg and repeat.

Alternate flex your right thigh with your left thigh five times.

Now flex both thighs at the same time for a count of five times.

Learn more: The thigh has three sets of strong muscles: the hamstring muscles in the back of the thigh, the quadriceps muscles in the front, and the adductor muscles on the inside. The quadriceps muscles and hamstring muscles work together to straighten (extend) and bend (flex) the leg. The adductor muscles pull the legs together.

Fidget #3: Tense your tummy:

Your abdominal muscles can be tensed if you are sitting or standing. Pull in your tummy and sit or stand up straight. Pay extra attention to your lower abdomen and squeeze those muscles hard.

Even if you're in a meeting, you can do this without anyone noticing.

Learn more: The abdominal muscles are a group that works together in three layers to provide support for your spine, assist in your breathing process, hold your organs in place and help with regulating internal abdominal pressure. Keeping your abdominal muscles toned is critical for your overall health, which is why so many exercise programs focus on them as your "core". The abdominal muscles are: external oblique, internal oblique, transverse abdominus, rectus abdominus and pyramidalis muscle.

Fidget #4: Advanced tummy roll:

This is hard to describe but think about forming an internal figure eight with your upper and lower abdominal muscles. I pull in my lower and push out my upper abs at the same time. Then reverse, pulling in the upper abdomen while relaxing the lower. It takes some practice but eventually it feels like a rolling figure eight, cycling up and down your abdomen.

Learn more: The so-called six-pack muscle is the rectus abdominus, which runs along the front of your tummy. Rolling your tummy deeply reaches the underlying transverse abdominus. Both are necessary for a toned midsection.

Fidget #5: Flex your calves:

The muscles at the back of your legs can be tensed without lifting your knees so it's an ideal hidden exercise to do anytime you are sitting.

Sit up straight in your chair. Flexing your calves is easier if you're not leaning back.

Flex your right calf then your left calf five times.

Flex both your calves together five times.

Learn more: Your calf is actually three separate muscles: gastrocnemius, soleus, plantaris and tibialis posterior. When you flex while sitting, the gastrocnemius and soleus engage. You can amplify their engagement by rising up on your toes. Doing this standing is a good way to develop your calf muscles as it engages all of them.

Fidget #6: Wiggle your feet:

Alternate lifting your toes and heels. Your knees will also lift so this is a more noticeable exercise. If you're sitting alone at a computer, watching television or in a dark movie house, keeping your feet moving will also help your blood flow in your lower legs.

Toe and heel lifts while sitting: You can work up good dance moves here! Pretend you're tapping to a rhythm.

Knee lift and foot circles: Lift each leg 4" off the floor. Circle your foot, paying attention to your ankles to make a smooth, even movement. Circle to the left five times then to the right five times.

Learn more: The foot has many muscles but an especially important one is the tibialis anterior, which runs to the shin. Tapping your toe helps keep strong which is vital for your ability to walk without falling. Calf muscles are often stronger than the tibialis anterior in the shin. Doing repeated toe tapping helps correct this muscle imbalance.

Fidget #7: Vaginal Kegels:

Every woman should be familiar with exercising her pelvic floor. The benefits for your sex life and also your urinary control are well-known and indisputable. If you are not doing kegels now, it's easy to start right now! You can flex the muscles in your vagina sitting, standing or laying down and no one will know but you. It's the perfect private fidget.

Just squeeze your vaginal muscles. If you can, try to identify the subtle differences from squeezing hard, from the front or deeper inside.

If you are at all shy about doing kegels, consider doing some research online. You will find an endless stream of encouraging articles with detailed directions.

Learn more: It's the puboccocygeus muscles of the pelvic floor that are tightened while doing kegels. Strengthening these muscles has multiple benefits including tightening the vagina, improving the control for urinary incontinence and preventing uterine prolapse. Men can also do kegels also which are used for treating prostate pain and urinary incontinence.

Fidget #8: Shoulder rolls:

This is the most obvious of my favorite fidgets. If there are people around, they are sure to notice that you are rolling your shoulders. It will be up to you to pick the best time and place, but shoulder rolls have great benefits. It's a great tension release, helps improve posture and makes your upper back and neck stronger.

Either standing or sitting, pull both shoulders up then push them back and roll forward to create a smooth circular motion.

Roll both shoulders together five times going back first. Then reverse direction and go forward first. The best form is to pull your shoulders up before circling front or back.

Roll your right and left shoulder separately five times.

Learn more: The shoulder roll motion involves a complex system of many muscles across the shoulder, upper chest and upper back. The deltoids, which run at the top of the arm into the upper chest and back. The trapezius are triangular muscles on each side of the upper back which run from the neck, across the shoulder blades down to the spine. The levator scapulae, which are located on both sides of the neck at the back and sides, assist lifting your shoulders.

Fidget #9: Hand and arm stretches, flaps and shakes:

Again, this fidget is hard to hide if you're out in public because it involves large arm movements. You could do some hand exercises under a table or desk but generally, I do arm movements when I'm in private. A good place is when you're in the bathroom! Just remember, ANY amount of time that you can keep moving will benefit to your weight control.

With your arms bent at the elbow, flap your arms out then back in. Do this ten times together then ten times with each arm separately.

Touch your shoulders then lift your arms straight up over your head. Bring them back down and touch your outer thighs. Do this ten times.

Make a fist and circle your wrist. Do both hands together five times then each hand separately five times.

There are many variations on arm and hand movements. Play around until you find a combination you enjoy.

In case you're curious: the arm and hands are a complicated system of muscles. The most well known are in your upper arm: the biceps in the front and the triceps at the back.

Learn more: The arm and hands are a complicated system of muscles. The biceps is actually two-headed muscle (biceps brachii) that shares its nerve supply with two other muscles in your forearm (brachialis and coracobrachialis). The rear arm muscle is called the deltoid. Lifting your arm sideways works the deltoid.

NO EXCUSES.
YOU CAN EXERCISE IN SO MANY DIFFERENT WAYS

Whether you walk around the block, sign up for a gym or follow a DVD at home, *if you want to control your weight, you must get moving.*

Exercise is big business. Even supermarkets sell yoga mats and exercise DVDs. It's hard to avoid the message that exercise is a necessary part of your day. Some of the marketing might be obnoxious, but it's also great reinforcement that everybody at every age can benefit from exercise.

Let yourself be reminded often that you need to keep moving. Park your car far away from the front door. Take the stairs. Leave your walking shoes out of the closet so you think of them often. If you have a friend to exercise with and support you, even better! Making agreements will help you stay on track.

If you sign up for a gym, consider one with scheduled classes. It's more powerful to have a time commitment and deadline to show up than a generalized "*I have to get to the gym*" frame of mind.

Personally, I've tried many different ways of exercising over the years and find that changing activities has been enjoyable. And sometimes necessary to keep me motivated. There have been times where I've shown up regularly at aerobics classes with a group, and other months when I start every day with a yoga DVD alone at home. These days I walk my dog every morning, swim about three times a week and use the weight machines at my gym twice a week.

Dancing is a way to combine exercise with joy. Professional dancers are incredible athletes, of course, but at whatever level you can dance, moving to music is a pleasure. You're very fortunate if this is a regular part of your life.

Even non-athletes can develop regular exercise habits and learn to love moving their bodies. It doesn't take long before you start to value and expect the extra movement in your life.

In my mind, a day without movement is a day I haven't taken good care of myself

Sure, some days my back hurts or I'm tired, but *there's no escape from the need to keep moving if I want to control my weight*. On the days that I haven't exercised, I know that it's important to get back to my regular schedule as soon as possible. Being sedentary is dangerous for me: my energy level drops and I notice more little aches and pains throughout my body.

Your self-respect will grow along with your increased ability to take care of your body. Moving for thirty minutes every day will be the cornerstone for building your healthy future.

Get started today!

HABIT #4
LEARN AND PRACTICE
PORTION CONTROL

Plan ahead and change visual cues
Set and accept limits

There are very few things more difficult in American life than accepting that we must set limits on what we can eat. Everywhere we turn there are advertisements for fast food, restaurants, sodas, candies. For those of us lucky enough to have money to spend, we can buy foods from all around the world, all year long around the clock.

We are taught that we can have it all, all the time.

It's easy to eat too much. American restaurant portions have grown dramatically over the last 20 years. Glasses are bigger, plates are larger and food is piled higher. "Supersize" is a word that didn't exist 25 years ago. (According to the Merriam-Webster Dictionary, the first known usage of "Supersize" was in 1994.) Now, it's such an ordinary word, everybody knows that it means bigger food portions.

Not only are we encouraged to eat more at meals, we're encouraged to eat more frequently. Snack food is big business selling billions of dollars each year, and the market is growing. The snack food industry works actively to blur the lines between meals by increasing the desire of target consumers (that would be you!) to eat more often. It's working!

How can you slow down this relentless rush to put more food in your mouth?

It's not easy, but it can be done. Let's take a look at some of the challenges you'll face learning portion control and how you can overcome them.

VISUAL CUES TELL YOU HOW MUCH TO EAT. CHANGE THE CLUES AND YOU GAIN CONTROL.

You will eat up to 30% more food if it's served in a big container. There's even a word for this: "Unit bias". This is the phenomenon of container size determining what we think the correct portion should be. Bigger dishes, taller cups, bigger boxes automatically trick us into eating bigger portions because we respond to visual cues for information about what's normal and right for us.

What we see sends stronger messages to our brain than the internal sensations from our stomachs.

Some cultures acknowledge this. For example, in Japan, there's an old saying that "We eat first with our eyes".

This is very important and should be repeated: *Your brain receives more information about what you should eat from your eyes than from your stomach.*

We are visually programmed to not feel full until the plate is empty. So, even though we've already eaten a full portion, if we still see a pile of food on the plate, we'll just keep eating.

Take control of your portions! Don't be tricked by the size of the plate into eating more than you should, if you're committed to controlling your weight. You have a powerful tool to help you, once you know how much what you see influences what you eat.

Start making changes by controlling the containers that serve your food.

- If you're home, use smaller bowls and plates.

- If you're at a restaurant which serves large portions, put an imaginary line down half the plate and ask for a doggie box. Then pack up half the meal to eat later.

- If you are getting take-out, don't eat directly out of the box. Putting the food on a plate, one portion at a time will help you stay in control.

- If you're buying a snack, don't eat directly out of the package. Put a portion in a small bowl.

- Pay attention to the size of the plate or container. Don't be passive if the portion is huge. You have the power to make changes and manage your portion size that sits in front of you.

- Make decisions about portion size BEFORE you start eating. This way you will be giving yourself valuable information and a strategy.

Take unneeded food off the table or put it away

Do you really need to eat bread and butter before your restaurant meal? Ask the waiter to remove the bread. Try it. Waiters do this all the time. You're not the only one asking.

Don't leave snacks laying out. Put all packages in cabinets or drawer. The exception to this is fruit. It's always smart to have a fruit bowl on your counter.

You've heard of the "See-Food Diet"? You see food then eat it? It's not a joke. Need proof? Think about the billions of dollars spent on advertising showing pictures of desirable food. Seeing food will make you yearn for it. If you don't parade temptations in front of your vision, you will be more successful controlling your cravings.

Avoid unconscious grazing. Pack up leftovers promptly.

If you're like me, it's easy to overeat at home because it's hard to stay out of the kitchen. I especially love to nibble on the food left around after a meal and need to force myself to put leftovers away quickly. If there are pots and plates of food left lying around, it's a tempting invitation.

Don't eat the leftovers from someone else's plate.

Nibbling while working in the kitchen while cleaning up didn't seem like so much food to me, but it adds up. There's something about not wanting to see food wasted that makes leftovers on plates so irresistible! But this becomes your second helping if you graze across the dinner plates and pans. For years, I struggled with unconsciously moving food into my mouth anytime I worked in the kitchen.

Avoiding eating after your meal should be finished takes a lot of discipline. It also takes storage containers, plastic wraps to cover bowls of leftovers, and a willingness to put food away for later.

Dedicate a cabinet to reusable storage containers that you can find in any grocery store, or reuse the containers from frozen food. I keep plastic wrap and rubber bands handy, also.

How big should a meal portion be?

How much you should eat at each meal is a complex question to answer since it depends on your body, your lifestyle and what kind of food you're eating. But, whether you snack all day long or eat separate meals, to control your weight you will have to pay attention to not eating more calories than your body burns.

The size of the portion isn't nearly as important as the type of food you've chosen. Visually, you could put a huge pile of lettuce on your plate and have fewer calories than 10 french fries.

Measuring portions by calories

Having an understanding of the calorie content of food is a critical skill for weight loss and weight control. You don't need to obsessively count calories, but you should be familiar with what adds calories to food and generally how much:

- Fat/oil is the most highly caloric substance we eat, at 9 calories per gram. One cupful of olive oil has 1,909 calories.

- Sugar and high fructose corn syrup are also very caloric. One cupful of sugar has 773 calories. One cupful of high fructose corn syrup has 871 calories.

There are many excellent calorie reference guides available that are lists of foods, a suggested portion and how many calories each portion contains. If you have no experience counting calories, I highly recommend that you buy one of these guides, and flip through it often. *The Calorie King® Calorie, Fat & Carbohydrate Counter* by Allan Borushek is a book available on Amazon, and for your smartphone, try the app *Calorie Counter & Diet Tracker* by My Fitness.

You can assign calorie totals to meals and snacks, based on how many calories you should be eating daily. Of course, your daily total will depend on whether you are trying to lose weight or maintain your existing weight. It will also vary depending on your age, size, exercise level, lifestyle and overall general health.

Here are recommendations for daily calorie intake from the US Health and Human Services and the US Department of Agriculture:

- 2,000 calories per day is the general recommendation for adult women to maintain weight. If you usually eat three meals a day, you could allow 500 calories per meal (for a total of 1,500 calories) and still have 500 calories left over for snacks and other eating.

- 2,500 calories per day is the general recommendation for adult men to maintain weight. If he usually eats three meals a day, he could have 600 calories per meal (for a total of 1,800 calories) and still have 700 calories left over for snacks and other eating. Yes, ladies, I agree that this is unfair!

You see how this formula works for portion control.

Calories are a large and important topic which we will discuss in more depth in *Habit #5: Know What's in Your Food Before You Put It in Your Mouth*. Be sure to read that chapter for more information.

Hate counting calories? Me, too. Here's what you can do instead.

If you hate counting calories, you could switch away from high-calorie foods like meat, cheese, sweets, butter or anything fatty, and chose to eat foods that provide a lot of volume and nutrition for relatively few calories. These wonder foods include vegetables, fruit, whole grains and legumes. You will be able to relax and not worry about counting calories for every meal.

In other words: If you eat cheeseburgers, you will need to pay constant attention. If you eat a plant-based diet, you can relax.

High-calorie foods, either because they contain a lot or sugar or a lot of fat are often referred to as "calorie dense foods". After a while, you will become practiced and very skilled at identifying what is a calorie dense food. For your weight control practices, it's best to restrict these to very small portions, or avoid them entirely.

Your portions can be larger if you stay away from calorie dense foods

If you're someone who loves mouth action—and I definitely love mouth action—staying away from calorie dense foods is the perfect solution. You can chew piles and piles of most vegetables and not really have to think very much about portion control. In fact, if you eat a vegetable salad with very little or no oil dressing, you can eat baskets full. I eat as many salads as I want, whenever I want, and load them with a variety of green, red and yellow vegetables. But I don't top the salads with cheese, croutons, lots or dressing, or top the vegetable dishes with butter or rich sauces.

Visually, it's not the square inches of the portion that matters. It's how dense the calorie content is. You could put a huge pile of green beans on your plate and have fewer calories than 10 French fries.

Practice measuring and weighing your food to learn portion size

Do you know what a cup of rice or pasta looks like on a plate? How about three ounces of chicken? Or two teaspoons of salad dressing? Knowing how to connect standard measurements like cupfuls with calories is a very important skill for portion control.

If you don't own measuring cups and measuring spoons, buy inexpensive sets and spend thirty minutes measuring what you have in the kitchen to become familiar with what 1 tablespoon, 1/4 cup, 1/2 cup and 1 cup portions look like. That way, you will know how much food to put on your plate.

Kitchen scales to measure weight are a bit more expensive but there are $9.99 models available on Amazon and in discount stores. Practice weighing meat and cheese until you are familiar with one, two and three ounce portions. Knowing portion sizes of calorie-dense and high-fat foods is very important for weight control.

Don't forget beverages! You're probably already familiar with the size of your glasses, and beverage containers are already marked but be extra careful with wine. We'll cover beverages more carefully in the section *Habit #6: Avoid Added Sugars and Sweetened Drinks.*

Mouthfuls matter. It's a small portion and you can savor the flavors.

Consider measuring in mouthfuls. One mouthful is about one tablespoon of volume, or the equivalent of 1/2 ounce. (Don't cheat by taking huge bites!)

This is useful for calorie dense foods that are full of fats and sugars. You need to be very disciplined with these and train yourself to think in small portions. A mouthful of chocolate cake may not seem like a reasonable portion now, but if you want to control your weight for the rest of your life and not give up treats, measuring by mouthfuls is a practical guideline.

Learn to eat treats by the mouthful, not the plateful and you won't need to worry about counting calories.

Give up treats for life? No! Eat them ONLY when you dine out and can share

Rich foods that give you pleasure, like chocolate or ice cream, can be part of your life if you master portion control. But it will be safer if you don't bring tempting treats into your home! Save the cake, candy, cookies and ice cream for when you're out.

Sharing a dish with a friend is a good technique. For example, when I go out to dinner with family or friends, we frequently order a single dessert to share. One spoonful of chocolate cake is enough to fill my mouth and keep me happy. I don't talk while I savor the flavors and take a long time to enjoy this treat.

The most rich, high-calorie foods can be enjoyed in small portions.

Recommended portion for cake and ice cream: One to three mouthfuls maximum.

That's right. At the most, only three mouthfuls. Make them count by eating very slowly and take plenty of time to enjoy every lick. You'll be surprised at how long a bite can last and how satisfying eating this way can be.

Don't torture yourself if it's just too tempting to have rich, sweet food available under any circumstances. If you can't limit yourself to one, two or three mouthfuls, staying away from temptation is probably your best choice. <u>Don't buy temptations, don't order temptations, and try not to look at them.</u>

Be kind to yourself and don't ask for trouble.

Precooking dinners in larger batches helps with daily portion control

It's easy meal prep to arrange food on plates from main dishes that are pre-cooked. This gives you greater control about portion size because you can control what's on your plate and put away the rest of the main dish for later.

I practice this at home by pre-cooking the main dish in large batches maybe twice a week, but almost always on Sunday. The main dish is usually what we eat for protein: chicken, a bean casserole, fish, tofu. Because our meals also include a lot of fresh vegetables, I expect to slice up a selection of vegetables to put on the plate, possibly after a quick pass on the stove in a pan with a little olive oil.

For a working parent, having food made in advance is a major time saver! And for those of you who love to cook, you can get all the action you want working with beautiful seasonal vegetables.

We live in a golden age of cooking with unprecedented access to ingredients. There are inspiring recipes to be had at the click of the computer. If you love to cook, you are used to measuring ingredients. Apply your good experience to measuring out reasonable meal portions.

WHEN DO YOU FEEL FULL? WHY YOUR STOMACH'S MESSAGE IS SLOW TO REACH YOUR BRAIN

It's sad but true—your stomach will not keep you informed in a timely manner that it's full. This is because humans do not have the internal nerve connections for very finely tuned awareness of our digestive activity.

The communication system between your digestive system and your conscious brain is complex but it doesn't always work quickly. Generally, it takes 20 minutes for your brain to register that your stomach has had enough to eat. In that 20 minutes, you can certain swallow a lot of food, well in excess of what would be a healthy, controlled portion.

This 20-minute communication gap is the source of many people's overeating.

For those of you who are curious about details, here is what happens: The vagus nerve connects the brain and stomach and is stimulated when your digestive track releases cholecystokinin, a peptide usually called CCK. It's CCK that carries the message to your brain that your stomach is full. The twenty minute delay is because CCK isn't released instantly. Food has to travel and be processed first.

Because visual clues already confuse us about how much to eat, a delay in feeling full really complicates matters. It's no wonder that we don't know when to stop eating.

BUT, now that you know, there are things you can do about it.

Eating more slowly will give your brain a chance to catch up

Try not to "inhale" your food. It will be very helpful if you can slow down the first ten minutes of eating. Try chewing your food more thoroughly. Finish each mouthful and swallow before you put more food in your mouth.

4 TIPS TO SLOW DOWN YOUR EATING	
Tip #1	Take smaller bites. Put less food on your fork or in your mouth.
Tip #2	Chew each bite very thoroughly and don't rush to swallow.
Tip #3	Take a sip of water inbetween each bite. Drinking fluid adds more volume to your stomach and helps you feel full faster.
Tip #4	Put the fork down after each bite. Wait for a count of five before you pick it up again.

Have a small appetizer to jumpstart your stomach's message

There are tricks you can use even before you sit down to eat a meal.

Since you're looking to bridge that 20 minute delay between your stomach and your brain, having a small appetizer before your meal is useful, especially if you're sitting down to a big dinner. You'll jumpstart your stomach's messaging and be inclined to eat less of the main meal because you'll feel full sooner. Olives or crunching fresh vegetables like carrots is a good idea. If cheese and crackers are your appetizer, be extra careful! Eating calorie-rich cheese is a quick way to put on extra pounds.

Drink a glass of warm water before the meal. It will help your brain get the message that your stomach is full.

Avoid filling up with bread and butter at a restaurant. Those are empty calories that will do nothing but sabotage your weight control efforts.

Pay extra attention to your internal clues

This is easier said than done! In our country, this is especially challenging because so many people eat surrounded by external distractions. We eat in front of the television, while driving in cars, or while focusing on our smart phones.

Try eating a meal with your eyes closed. Eating while tuning in to your sensory responses requires slowing down and paying attention. See if you can savor every bite and feel the food traveling inside your body. You don't have to be a Zen master to be more in touch with your digestive system. Try it once. It's worth it!

Skipping a meal can lead to overeating next time. Don't skip meals!

Skipping meals prevents your metabolism from running smoothly. Your body needs energy to keep going. It will convert your food into sources of energy, primarily glucose in your blood stream, which a healthy metabolism uses up in about three hours. After that, your body draws on energy storage, primarily glycogen, a carbohydrate stored in your liver and muscles.

You may think that you're avoiding calories and pulling down your fat storage if you skip a meal, but really you're setting yourself up to feel so uncomfortable with low blood sugar that you could easily grab too much food the next time you have a chance.

Eating regularly is the best way to make sure that you're not desperately hungry at a meal and overeat

Drinking wine or beer? Alcohol affects your self-control

Impairing your judgment and self-control is a well-known side effect of drinking any kind of alcohol. If you have one or more drinks with your meal, your self-control will be seriously affected, making it much harder for you to set limits.

Keep this in mind, especially if you are eating a meal with cheese or fried foods. These are the most dangerous, calorie-laden foods that require masterful portion control. Your ability to avoid them or only eat just three mouthfuls will seem laughable after a couple of beers.

Before you start drinking, plan your meal sensibly. Know in advance what you will eat and what you can't touch.

FAT IS NOT TOXIC. WE NEED IT TO SURVIVE, BUT PORTION CONTROL IS CRITICAL.

Your body requires fat to stay healthy. It uses fat to build new cells, keep your organs healthy, insure that they're working properly, and regulate your hormones. Without fat, your metabolism can't properly use many vitamins and minerals. It's absolutely essential to eat some fat in your diet.

But fat is the most calorie dense food on Earth. There is no other food that packs as many calories in each mouthful. All fats (vegetable oils, animal fat, butter, etc.) have approximately 9 calories per gram. That's about 35 calories per teaspoon, or 105 calories in every tablespoon. One cupful has a staggering 1,909 calories.

Learning portion control for fats is a critical skill because nothing will damage your quest for weight control faster than extra fat calories sneaking into your daily eating. The question is how much—and which kind of fat—should you eat regularly. You probably already know that fats from animals and fats found in plants are different in their health benefits or risks. (Think about lard from beef compared to olive oil.)

There is a more detailed discussion about dietary fats in *Habit #5: Know What's in the Food You Eat Before You Put it in Your Mouth.*

Here are some simple portion guidelines you can follow for fats:

- Limit oils to one teaspoon per portion. If you are pan-frying anything, don't use more than this. If the food in the pan is for four people, you can use four teaspoons. You will be surprised at how well just a little oil will cook food.

- Limit butter to one teaspoon per meal. If you use butter to fry eggs, one teaspoon is more than enough for two eggs. If you eat bread, try putting on only a thin film of butter. You'll still get the flavor.

- Butter substitutes are very useful. For cooking on the stovetop, I prefer a butter-tasting vegetable oil spread from Brummel & Brown. It tastes good and has only 15 calories per teaspoon.

- Avoid fried foods. Oils are absorbed into the foods, especially porous vegetables like potatoes. One cup of french fries has 440 calories. The potato portion is only 150 calories. You're mostly eating oil!

- Eating meat? Stick with the leanest cuts and limit your portion to 3 ounces. That's about a half a cupful, if it were chopped up. Practice weighing your favorite cooked meats so you understand how much volume it takes to make a three ounce portion.

- Learn to limit salad dressings. Have them "on the side" and dip your fork into the dressing before loading it with salad. You'll get the flavor and almost none of the calories.

- If possible, learn to love salad without dressing. I love the crunch of lettuce and cucumber. If you can tolerate salt, that's a good substitute for oily dressings. If you buy oil-free dressings, watch out for their sugar content.

Think low-fat 2% milk gets 2% of the calories from fat? Think again!

The fat content is usually measured by weight, not by percentage of calories. This can be <u>so</u> misleading.

Low-fat 2% milk has 120 calories per 8 ounce glass. It contains 5 grams of fat which is measured by weight. We know that each gram of fat has 9 calories, so 8 ounces of this milk must have 9 x 5 = 45 calories from fat.

45 Calories is 37% of the 120 calorie total.

Confused? Me, too. This is why some food labels are now required to include the actual number of calories from fat, not just the gram count. Most consumers are too busy trying to rush through the store to read labels. But if you want to master weight control, you need to understand what's in the food you're eating.

To master portion control, get in the habit of reading nutrition labels

Reading nutrition labels is a critical skill for weight control. This can't be stressed enough. If you buy and eat packaged foods without reading the nutrition label for fat and sugar content, you are "shooting yourself in the foot" and will make weight control efforts more difficult. Eating hidden fats and sweeteners is easy to do, especially if your day includes processed foods.

KEEPING A FOOD DIARY HELPS WITH PORTION CONTROL

Few tips or practices are as universally applauded for weight loss success as keeping a food diary. Writing down everything you eat and drink has many benefits including being able to be realistic about what has gone into your mouth.

I have found that keeping a food diary is very helpful in keeping the weight off, also, especially during times when temptation seems to be all around. I don't always keep a food diary, but it is a practice that I resume anytime my resolve to resist empty calories is starting to slip.

Writing everything down is a deterrent to eating unconsciously, especially if you really lean in and honestly write down everything you've eaten or had to drink. Even that mouthful of cookie which jumped into your mouth. If you're like me, you will find that your careless eating and drinking habits clean up when you carry a food diary notebook all the time.

It doesn't need to be fancy. You can buy a pocket notebook for $2.00, then if something enters your mouth, a notation needs to enter the book.

Here's what to write:

- What the food or drink is. (Ex: apple, coffee with 2% milk, chicken without skin.)

- The quantity you ate or drank. (Ex: apple: ½ ; coffee: 6 oz cup; chicken 3 oz.)

- Enter your estimate of the calories if you're actively trying to loose weight.

- For weight loss, add up your calories in the morning and at the start of the evening. That way, you'll know how much you can still eat for the day. (Your weight loss should have a target, possibly 1,500 calories per day. Please check with your doctor.)

- Write down any useful tips you learn during the day. You can also write affirmations and encouraging statements which you will see and read repeatedly. This can help you stay inspired and on track for the day.

MASTERING PORTION CONTROL IS A MAJOR LIFE SKILL

There's no point in pretending that learning to master portion control is easy. It's not. All around us there are encouragements to overeat and eat frequently. And, our biology doesn't help by being designed to be so responsive to what we see. Our long-ago ancestors, before agriculture was invented, only ate if they could find or hunt for food, so it helped their survival if they could gorge themselves whenever there was an opportunity.

The trouble is that some of us still love to gorge ourselves. I love overeating. I love chewing and swallowing and having my stomach feel full. I truly understand the desire to do so. But, over the years, I learned to love my health and my slim figure more, and accepted that my eating must have limits. I resent having limits, but I know that I must honor them if I don't want to gain weight.

It's very, very difficult to value an abstract idea like good health over the concrete reality of that juicy 8 oz steak and pile of French fries in front of you.

One last piece of advice: try to surround yourself with people who do not have an overeating problem. Eat meals with them and carefully observe what they do. Take mental notes and try to copy their good habits. Not everyone struggles with portion control. Some people are naturally able to eat wisely. Do you best to become one of them.

For extra help with learning to control food cravings, see *Habit #10: Learn to Control Your Food Cravings: Ways to deal with excessive food desire and get help when you need it.*

HABIT #5
KNOW WHAT'S IN YOUR FOOD
BEFORE YOU PUT IT IN YOUR MOUTH

Learn about calories, fats and carbohydrates
The Glycemic Index

Calories, fats and carbohydrates are enormously complicated subjects and hard to simplify because there is so much information. Let's start at the beginning with basic descriptions of what calories are.

WHAT IS A CALORIE?

Calories-in: Simply put, a calorie is the way scientists measure the energy contained in food. Sometimes the word "energy" is replaced by the words "work" or "heat" or even "heat energy". To be more precise, scientists calculate small calories—with a lower-case "c"—as the amount of energy required to raise one gram of water one degree celsius. A large calorie—with a capital "C"—is the amount of energy required to raise one kilogram of water one degree celsius.

When it comes to measuring calories in food, scientists use the small "c" calorie, so even if this sounds complicated, it's easy to compare foods because the unit of measurement is the same. Calories in food are a measurement of the units of energy that food will provide.

When food labels list calories, they offer a guideline using measurements like cupfuls or ounces or grams. Don't get confused. Be observant if you are comparing calories and make sure that your units of measurement are the same. That way, it's easy to see that different foods have different calorie totals for the same measurement.

Here are two extreme examples:

- A cupful of olive oil has 1,909 calories but a cupful of chopped carrots has 52 calories.

- A cupful of sugar has 774 calories but a cupful of cooked oatmeal without sugar has 158 calories.

Trying to keep an accurate calorie count of what you're eating can be confusing because most of the foods you are eating are blends of different ingredients, even a simple blend like cheese on a cracker. This is especially true whether you cook your meals or buy your meals at a restaurant.

I am not an advocate of obsessively counting calories, although I have done that in the past, but I do believe that if you want to control your weight for life, it's a requirement to invest some effort into learning more about what you're eating. It's vitally important to be curious about what you're putting in your body!

Calories-out: Your body uses energy as it lives through the day, and "calorie" is the unit that scientists use to measure how much energy has been used. You're familiar with the phrase "calories burned" by exercise. It means the same as "calories out".

Here are examples:

- An hour of moderate walking burns about 255 calories.

- An hour of jumping rope burns 1,074 calories.

- Just sitting in your chair burns about 84 calories per hour.

Here's why it matters that you understand about calories

Not all calories are processed the same way by your metabolism, as we will see later in this chapter. A calorie is not a calorie when it comes from different types of foods like proteins or carbohydrates. But total calories still count.

If you eat more calories than your body burns, you will gain weight. Simple. If you move around a lot, you can eat more and either maintain your weight or lose some pounds. If you spend most of your time sitting and don't restrict how many calories you eat, you will get heavier.

Calories-In / Calories-Out must be in balance for your weight to be maintained. To lose weight, you need to both increase your movement throughout the day and make smarter calorie choices about what you are putting in your mouth.

Do you really need to memorize calorie numbers? Yes, but just these two.

Here's the most important number you need to memorize:

- The average adult woman needs 2,000 calories daily, based on moderate activity. (If you're a man, the average number is 2,500 calories daily, based on moderate activity.)

The number most commonly referred to for all adults is 2,000 calories. (On nutrition labels, you'll read the statement: "Percentage Daily Values are based on a 2,000 calorie diet".) Age, gender, size and activity level make a difference, of course, but 2,000 calories daily is a good basic number.

Here's the second important number you need to know:

- Each pound of fat on your body is worth 3,500 calories.

That means that if you eat 3,500 calories more than you burn over the course of seven days, you will gain one pound that week. That's why weight creeps up on you. You don't have to overeat gross amounts every day. Just a little bit of overeating will add the pounds over time.

That's also the good news: just small adjustments in what you're eating will reduce your incoming calories over the weeks and the weight will fall off gradually.

You will lose weight by reducing your daily calories

You can steadily lose weight by reducing your daily calorie intake to less than 2,000 calories per day.

When I've been on a vacation and have gained a few pounds, I reduce my calorie intake by 25% from the recommended daily total of 2,000 and rigorously follow the 10 Daily Habits. This means that I'm careful not to eat more than 1,500 calories a day, while still being careful that my meals and snacks are nutritious. With 30 minutes of daily exercise, you'll lose about two pounds a week following this guideline.

I've been on medicially supervised liquid diets that only allow 600 calories daily. The weight dropped off, but, of course, it flooded back on when I stopped the program.

Detox programs, fasts, quick weight loss diets that promise you'll drop 10 or 20 pounds in a month, all rely on calorie reduction, no matter what they recommend you eat.

Removing a pound of fat, with its 3,500 calories, from your body, is a complex process that can be influenced by many factors of your individual biochemistry. There may be metabolic factors at play which make it difficult for your body to shed weight. But, in general, most people will lose weight reducing calories while following what the 10 Daily Habits offers: a low-carb, low-fat, low-sugar and high-fiber lifestyle diet.

Should you count calories every day?

If you are just learning about calorie content in foods, then yes, I recommend that you invest in a calorie book, be prepared to write down what you're eating, and make the effort to count all calories you eat from the time you wake up until the time you go to sleep.

Why? To control your weight, you need to learn about your food environment. You need to understand as much as possible about what you're putting in your mouth. Remember, you are working on creating a permanent lifestyle, not a quick weight-loss diet. You can expect to invest some time learning how to do it. Put in a little work learning about the calorie content of the foods you eat and you will have the knowledge for the rest of your life.

Here's what you need:

- A portable source of information, either a small calorie counter book or an app for your phone.

The book I recommend is: *The Calorie King® Calorie, Fat & Carbohydrate Counter* by Allan Borushek, available on Amazon and at www.calorieking.com. This is also available for Kindle, IPod and IPhone.

- The smartphone app I recommend is: *Calorie Counter & Diet Tracker* by My Fitness.

If you are an experienced calorie counter, but have "fallen off the wagon" and gotten out of the habit of paying attention, then maybe you just need a few days of counting to jumpstart your memory.

Should you keep a food diary and write down your calories? Yes!!

The practice of keeping a daily food dairy is widely supported by doctors, nutrition specialists and weight loss professionals. An amazing study of 1,700 dieters found that those who kept track of what they ate lost twice as much as those people who didn't. (Weight Loss Maintenance Trial Research Group, Kaiser Permanente Center for Health Research. 2008)

Those dieters lost twice as much with a food dairy!

Keeping a food diary means that you write down everything you eat. Everything. It will force you to be mindful about what you're putting in your mouth. If you eat without paying much attention, this is a discipline that will be hugely beneficial for you. If you're trying to lose weight, why wouldn't you want to use a tool that will double your weight loss for the same amount of effort?

When my eating habits start becoming careless, keeping a food diary puts me back on track. I carry a food diary notebook in my purse and am constantly reminded of my goals to practice healthy eating habits which promote weight control.

For much more information on keeping a food diary, see *Bonus Habit #2: Keep a Food Diary.*

Paying attention isn't always easy, so don't forget to find a moment at the end of the day to praise yourself for your efforts. Reflect on what you've eaten. Congratulate yourself if you've stayed on target, and resolve to do better tomorrow if you've strayed.

You can track calories-in easily, but can you track calories-out?

I don't think tracking calories-out is a practical goal. You don't have the equipment that scientists have to measure movement, expiration, and all the metrics used to determine how much energy a body is actually using.

Calories-in are easy to track if you keep to the stated portion (in ounces, grams, cupfuls) because many years of scientific measurements have gone into developing those numbers, which are now printed for you to read.

So, don't use average activity numbers and subtract them from your daily calorie totals.

I recommend that you <u>don't think about the calories you are burning as a savings account you can draw down on and spend by eating more</u>.

The goal is to make daily exercise part of your life, a part that feels so natural that you don't need to treat it a something special with special rules. Exercising every day is a primary health and weight management strategy. If you start using exercise as a way to justify having treats you will sabotage your long-term efforts to control your weight.

If you are really curious and wish to have more accurate information about how many calories you are burning while you exercise, ask your doctor for a recommendation to a respected nutritionist who will be able to guide you.

HIGH CALORIE = CALORIE DENSE IT'S THE SAME MEANING. HERE'S WHY UNDERSTANDING MATTERS SO MUCH TO YOU

High calorie and calorie dense are the same terms for food that is packed with calories. This also means that it is low in water and fiber content, because the density of food material is affected by how much water and fiber it contains. Water content doesn't need to be dripping or visually obvious. It could be in food like broccoli, which is very solid but contain a lot of water in its structure. Fiber is also something you can't see with the naked eye.

Calorie dense food is usually very high in fat and/or carbohydrates. Since sugar is the best known carbohydrate. Here's an interesting contrast:

- 1 Cup of sugar has 774 calories.

- 1 Cup of broccoli has 31 calories

- 1 Cup of water has 0 calories

- 1 Cup of psyllium husks has 132 calories. (High fiber powder like Meta-mucil used by many people for regularity.)

Thinking about calorie density is a new way to think about food for most of us. What I really like about thinking about food as "calorie dense" instead of "high calorie" is that it forces you to think about the food's internal structure. This is extremely useful and puts you in the mindset of being ready to learn more about what's inside the food you're eating.

Having an understanding about why food is calorie-dense will help you control your weight.

Eat mostly foods that are not calorie dense and limit portion sizes of calorie-dense foods very carefully.

It's not hard to learn—you already know that foods differ wildly in how many calories each mouthful contains. Just think about which food has more water and fiber, and which has more fat and added sugars. When you start thinking about calorie density of any type of food, you will have a valuable key to portion control, which is a primary skill necessary for your weight control lifestyle.

Cheese, for example, is calorie dense and has more calories per mouthful than apples because cheese is almost entirely fat with very little water and no fiber. Apples are full of water, have fiber and no fat. Chocolate is usually high in both fat and sugar, but contains no fiber and little water.

Here are charts for you with suggested portions. Limit the calorie dense food according to the chart below, and don't overeat! If you can't resist, consider avoiding the calorie dense foods until your habit of portion control is more established.

These lists are intended to offer guidelines of which types of foods are very calorie dense. As such, I've used averages of foods like cheese, cake and ice cream. For more accurate calorie, fat and sugar information about a specific food, please check one of your calorie counter books or apps.

CALORIE DENSITY IN COMMON FOODS
Try to eat foods that are not calorie dense

HIGH CALORIE-DENSE FOODS: CAREFULLY LIMIT YOUR PORTIONS OR AVOID

FOOD	PORTION	CALORIES	HIGH IN FAT OR ADDED SUGAR?
Cheese (Average of all types)	1 oz	110	Yes: Fat
Beef (steak, hamburger not lean)	4 oz	380	Yes: Fat
Fried foods (fried chicken)	4 oz	320	Yes: Fat
Butter	1 tbsp	100	Yes: Fat
Oil	1 tbsp	120	Yes: Fat
Mayonnaise	1 tbsp	90	Yes: Fat
Nuts (Average of all types)	¼ cup	180	Yes: Fat, some fiber
Sugar	1 tbsp	46	Yes: Sugar
High fructose corn syrup	1 tbsp	53	Yes: Sugar
Bread (heavy, whole grain)	1 slice	110	Possibly fat & sugar
Pastry (bear claw)	3 oz	540	Yes: Fat and sugar
Donut (glazed)	3 oz	320	Yes: Fat and sugar
Cakes (chocolate)	3 oz	300	Yes: Fat and sugar
Cookies (chocolate chip)	1.5 oz	80	Yes: Fat and sugar

Chocolate	1 oz	150	Yes: Fat and sugar
Ice cream (vanilla)	3 oz	175	Yes: Fat and sugar
Wine	4 oz	100	Yes: Sugar
Beer	12 oz	140	Yes: Sugar
Distilled spirits	2 oz	130	Sugar

MODERATELY CALORIE DENSE FOODS: EAT MORE OF THESE

FOOD	PORTION	CALORIES	HIGH IN FAT OR ADDED SUGAR?
Beans (dried, cooked)	1 cup	210	No
Whole grains (average, cooked)	1 cup	175	No
Corn	1 cup	160	No
Potatoes and starchy vegetables (hold the butter)	1 cup	180	No
Bread (light, whole grain)	1 slice	50	Possibly fat & sugar
Tortilla wrap (average)	1 wrap	90	Possibly fat & sugar
Chicken (without skin)	3 oz	165	No
Fish (without sauce or oil)	3 oz	108	No
Eggs	2 eggs	140	No
Yogurt (plain, unsweetened)	½ cup	70	No

NOT CALORIE DENSE FOODS:
EAT UNLIMITED AMOUNTS OF GREEN, RED & ORANGE VEGETABLES

FOOD	PORTION	CALORIES	HIGH IN FAT OR SUGAR?
Green, red vegetables	1 cup	30	No
Fruit (average)	1 piece	100	No
Condiments	1 tsp	25	Mixed. Use common sense.

There are many different approaches to categorizing food. Calorie density is my personal favorite, but I'm not a diabetic who needs to count carbohydrate grams. The best way of categorizing and ranking food according to carbohydrate content is the **Glycemic Index.** Please see the section on carbohydrates in this chapter for more information.

WHAT ARE "EMPTY CALORIES"?

An "empty calorie" is what you get when you eat or drink something that has no beneficial nutrition to give your body. The nutrition value is zero.

For example, if you drink a 12-ounce can of Pepsi, you consume 150 calories but there isn't anything nutritious that your body can actually use except the water content. The 150 calories come from sugar (or high fructose corn syrup) in sodas. You can live very nicely without sugar so these are 150 do-no-good calories. Another example is the candy bar I used to love as a child: Nestlé's Butterfinger Bar. One king-size bar has 495 calories. As a teenager, I would eat one of these daily. No wonder my weight ballooned to 220 pounds.

ChooseMyPlate.gov is very clear about daily limits for empty calories:

- For women 31 – 50 years: No more than 160 empty calories per day. (The equivalent of 10 teaspoons of added sugar.)

- For men 31 – 50 years: No more than 265 empty calories per day. (The equivalent of 17 teaspoons of added sugar.)

It's easy to add empty calories to your day. From sugary morning cereals with false promises about being "fortified" and "healthy", to colorful bags of chips and counters full of candy bars, it's just hard to avoid seeing the vast quantities of empty calories all around us. Temptation seems to be everywhere. And, if we go to restaurants, there's always the offer of dessert. Many of us grew up having dessert with dinner every night at home so we want to end our meal with a sweet. Well, that sweet is empty calories.

Here are the dominant sources of empty calories you should avoid:

- **Sodas with sweeteners:** These are sweetened and flavored water and are targeted as main culprits for the obesity epidemic. When I drank sodas, I drank Diet Pepsi and avoided the calories from sweeteners. If you must drink sodas, chose the ones that are artificially sweetened. (And be aware that you're pouring chemicals in your body. Drinking water is really a better idea.)

- **Juices with sweeteners:** Beware of the now trendy juice drinks that are loaded with added sweeteners. Read the labels carefully.

- **Coffee drinks:** Who doesn't love those fancy Starbucks coffees, topped with whipped cream and drizzled with syrup? The calorie load is stupendously out of proportion for the little bit of calcium and protein you get from the milk.

- **Chips:** We all love to crunch, but whether the chips are fried or baked, they're still empty calories. Don't buy bags of chips, including packaged vegetable chips which are very high in fat. For optimal weight control, crunch on fresh carrot or cucumber slices instead.

- **Candy:** It doesn't matter what you read about the benefits of dark chocolate. These are marginal compared to the empty calories you'll be taking in. Don't put temptation in your path by having candy at home. If you must see it at work, imagine that it's a bowl of worms. Consider that candy bars in stores are completely off limits. At social gatherings, if you can't hold yourself to one or two mouthfuls, don't get started at all.

- **Cakes and cookies:** We love baked goods. And they can be so lovely and appealing! They're high in sugar and fat, which is not going to help you control your weight. Watching other people eat cakes and cookies is especially difficult. Give yourself an alternate action with your mouth. If it's impolite to chew gum, sip on coffee, tea or water.

- **Fried foods:** Whether it's fried chicken, tempura vegetables, French fries, donuts or churros, you don't need that much fat from oils and grease. Many of the diet professionals I worked with over the years banned fried foods entirely. Anything fried was completely forbidden. It's simple to know why: The act of frying absorbs more oil than you need. Stay away!

Read *Habit #10: Control Your Food Cravings* for helpful information on how you can resist temptation.

Let's admit that it's not easy to resist the temptation of empty calorie foods. That's why weight loss programs like Nutrisystem often feature desserts in their ads. The message is "You don't have to give up anything". Well, it's time for a reality check. If you want to lose and *control* your weight after you've lost it, you must be prepare to limit or give up certain types of foods. And, at the top of that list are foods with empty calories.

But what about pleasure?
Do we always need to think about what the food contains and what's offered for nutrition?

Beautiful, well-prepared food is indeed a pleasure, and it's too bad that we need to be so analytical. If you have struggled with extra pounds on your body and you wish to control your weight at a healthy, lower level, then you simply need to understand what's in the food you eat. Sorry, but yes, you do need to be analytical and aware of the food's content.

You can surrender to pleasure *after* you've considered the food and carefully measured out your portion.

A large part of the pleasure I receive from eating and cooking food is looking at the beautiful ingredients. When shopping, I head first for the produce section, and if the store has made the effort to display fruits and vegetables nicely, I take a moment to enjoy their shapes and colors.

If I'm lucky to get to a farmer's market, admiring the bounty of what nature can provide us is a source of deep pleasure. I also love looking at bakery windows, ogling at cakes, cookies, pastries and the artistry of bakers. Food is wonderful. If we are so fortunate to live where we have many choices, just looking at them is a celebration.

Pleasure comes in many different ways, not just in your mouth. In *Habit #9: Enjoy at Least One Non-Caloric Pleasure Every Day,* we discuss how you can enhance receiving pleasure in your life.

ARE ALL CALORIES CREATED EQUAL? YES! NO! IT'S COMPLICATED!

A fierce debate is raging in the diet and nutrition world about whether the source of calories you eat makes a difference in weight control. One side says "yes": carbohydrate calories are used differently by our bodies than protein and fat calories. The other side says "no": calorie totals are what really count.

There is a famous story to prove that only the grand total of calories actually counts. A scientist went on a Hostess Twinkie diet, eating a Twinkie every 3 hours along with other sugary snacks. By reducing his overall daily calorie intake, he lost 27 pounds over 10 weeks. As a university professor, he had access to top health care to clean up any consequences from this crazy experiment. Don't try this at home!

So, here are basic biological truths:

- Eating excess calories will promote weight gain.
- Reducing calories to less than you are burning will promote weight loss.

The types of calories you eat will have a long-term impact on how well your metabolism will work over the years.

Calories, which do not contain nutrients, will leave you with the consequences of vitamin and mineral deficiencies. Calories, which are devoid of fiber, will digest quickly, breaking down into glucose faster than your metabolism can process it. Fiber slows down digestion. Without it—and refined white flour has been stripped of its fiber—your pancreas spikes too much insulin causing your blood sugar to drop too far. Short-term, you feel hungry again very soon. Long-term, your muscles start developing insulin resistance so the extra blood sugar is stored as fat.

Bottom line: refined white flour and sugars taste good but it aren't healthy for you. If it's a major part of your core diet, it's time for a change.

If you'd like to learn more, I recommend these well-respected books

- *Why Calories Count: From Science to Politics* by Marion Nestle and Malden Nesheim. This highly detailed book by two of America's most influential nutrition scientists will answer your questions about what calories are and what they do in our bodies.

- *Good Calories, Bad Calories: Challenging The Conventional Wisdom on Diet, Weight Control, and Disease* by Gary Taubes, an award-winning science journalist. Taubes states the case that the kind of calories we are eating makes a difference for our long-term health because carbohydrate calories affect the hormones which regulate insulin.

It's clear: overall calories must be controlled *and* what you eat makes a difference for how well your metabolism will work over the years.

LET'S TALK ABOUT DIETARY FAT: HERE'S WHAT YOU NEED TO KNOW

You could spend a lifetime studying fats and how they affect the human body and, in fact, many scientists and nutritionists do. It's a field that is expanding rapidly, with new findings that often contradict what our parents and grandparents believed.

For example, my father-in-law was a Type 1 diabetic, diagnosed at a young age. In the 1930's, doctors told him to eat more fats and oils, especially mayonnaise, because it would help control his diabetes. He dutifully started every day with a bowl of mayonnaise for breakfast. Can you imagine hearing that kind of medical advice today?

Here are current facts you need to know about dietary fat:

- Every living thing needs fat to function and survive. There is fat in the cells of everything that's alive, including plants like spinach.

- Your brain is 60% fat.

- Fat in your diet is absolutely essential because your body needs fat to build new cells, keep your organs healthy and working properly, maintain your nervous system, regulate your hormones and properly use many vitamins and minerals.

- No fat is water soluble, so your metabolism must take the extra step of breaking down all types of fat into fatty acids. Your system produces a special material called "lipoprotein" to carry the fat throughout your bloodstream.

- You are probably familiar with the most well known lipoproteins: LDL (low-density), HDL (high-density) and triglycerides, famous from cholesterol test results.

- If you eat more fat than your body can use immediately, it will be stored in fat cells (also called adipose cells) for future energy use. This is a complicated process. Removing fat from these cells is only done as your body's last resort, after all other sources of available energy are exhausted. (Ex: Glucose in your bloodstream. If you have available glucose circulating in your blood to use for energy and your metabolism will never dip into your fat cells and use up those reserves. Think about that before you put more sugar in your coffee!)

- All dietary fat is calorie dense. Fat is the most calorie dense food we ever eat. One gram is 9 calories. One tablespoon of oil or butter is about 120 calories.

- The words "fat" when they also mean "oil" are often interchangeable, especially in articles about health. All oils are types of fat so sometimes this can get confusing. (Olive oil is mostly monounsaturated fat. Canola oil is polyunsaturated fat.)

- Chefs and cookbook writers say "Fat is flavor". Humans love the taste of fatty foods. We also love sweet foods, which is why food that is processed to have its fat removed is often loaded with sweeteners instead. The result is that fat calories are just swapped for sweetener calories, sometimes with a total calorie gain! Yikes! Watch out for that when you reach for the "low-fat" food.

Here are the types of dietary fats you should be familiar with:

- **Saturated fats:** These are solid at room temperature and include all animal fats like cheese, butter, meat fats. A very few vegetable fats are solid: coconut and palm oil. Eating saturated fats is thought to raise your harmful cholesterol and increase inflammation and insulin resistance.

- **Unsaturated fats:** These are liquid at room temperature and mostly come from plants. Here's where is gets complicated. There are mono and poly types of saturated fats, depending on the source.

- **Monounsaturated fats**: These are available from vegetables, nuts and seeds including oils from olives, peanuts, canola.

- **Polyunsaturated fats**: These are also available from different vegetables, nuts and seeds including oils from corn, soybeans, sunflower, walnuts and fish. Omega-3 and Omega-6 fatty acids come from polyunsaturated fats.

- **Trans fatty acids:** These are naturally found in small quantities in meat and dairy, and man-made trans fats have been universally condemned as toxic. They are being legislated out of circulation as a public health issue.

It is popular today to advise avoiding the saturated fats from animals and it's fascinating to follow the debate and research about how much animal fat is healthy for humans to eat. Generally, Americans have received the message that high-fat diets of any kind are not healthy and we eat a lot less fat today (as a percentage of our calories) than our parents did. This seems hard to believe but it's true.

Our fat eating habits have changed over the years

When my mother was cooking my meals, the average American family got 45% of our calories from fats. Today, the average American diet is down to 30% fat calories. My mom didn't have access to fancy oils—even olive oil was considered fancy in the 1950's! She used Crisco and butter for cooking. We ate steak and didn't look at the food on our plate like a chemistry experiment. Yet, my parents were slender and I became fat. What happened?

I ate bigger portions. I loved chicken skin and drowned my salads in oily dressings. After dinner was over, my parents were finished eating for the night but I would reward myself with ice cream when my homework was finished. On the way home from school, I would spend my allowance on chocolate bars (50% or more calories from fat.) When I got home, I would have buttered toast before dinner. Things got really out of control when I left for college and could eat as much ice cream, pizza and chocolate as I wanted. My weight ballooned when I was a college freshman.

How much total fat you eat probably matters more than what kind

Your body absolutely needs fat in your diet to be healthy but if you look at the literature about what kind of fat to eat, your head will be spinning with confusion.

Generally, for many decades, most scientists have considered unsaturated fats from plants and fish to be healthier for you than saturated fats from animals. But, yes, you can find plenty of cases of groups of people who live happy, healthy lives eating cheese, butter and fatty meats. Think about the French, who eat a lot of cheese! Nutritionists call the heart-healthy, cheese-loving people in France who remain slender, the French Paradox.

The American Heart Association now recommends that all types of fats are no more than 25% of your total calories.

This is easy to explain, once you know about how to count calories:

If your daily calorie total is 2,000, no more than 500 calories should come from any type of fat.

See the American Heart Association website for more details at www.heart.org.

Personally, I think this is good advice. It avoids the issue of whether the fat is saturated or unsaturated, which I think is sensible, and only addresses your overall total of fat calories. For weight control, it's the grand total of your fat calories that will count.

If you eat a mostly plant-based diet, this is a very easy goal to accomplish. If your diet is filled with processed foods, meat, cheese and fried foods, you're going to have a hard time!

For weight control, it's all about making an informed choice and doing your best to stay away from high fat foods, whether they are saturated or unsaturated. When it comes to flooding your body with calories, they all have about 120 calories a tablespoon. Those calories add up very fast.

For a long time I tried to keep my daily fat calories to 25% of my daily total, and discovered immediately that it was easier to chose foods that were naturally low fat (like vegetables, whole grains, legumes and fruits) instead of having to calculate by portions. But some good foods are naturally high fat, so I exercised rigid portion control. Putting a tablespoon of olive oil on my salad, eating a ¼ cup of almonds, or enjoying a cupful of whole milk Greek yogurt gave me both the fat and the control I needed. Avoiding mayonnaise on sandwiches, reading all labels to look for hidden fats in breads or granola cereals, was all part of my 25% rule.

There are many ways to avoid fat, but the first is to understand how fat calories are reported on nutrition labels.

How to read nutrition labels for fat calories and percentages

Well, the labels don't make it easy, and they are often misleading, giving you a percentage next to fat content that is actually the percent of your "recommended daily allowance" of grams.

These days, fortunately, nutritionists managed to lobby the food label regulators to include calories from fat. But although listing <u>calories from fat</u> is now required for most nutrition labels, this does not tell you the <u>percentage fat calories are of the total</u>. The label can be confusing to understand if you are thinking in both absolute numbers and percentages at the same time.

Here is a simple formula that will help you! It can be done in seconds on your smart phone. With a little practice, it will be second nature and you'll never be confused again.

Step #1: On the nutrition label, look for the calories from fat per portion. Then look for the total calories in that portion.

Step #2: Divide the fat calories by the total calories.

Step #3: Move the decimal point two spaces to the right. That's your percentage!

Here are some examples:

FOOD AND PORTION	CALORIES	CALORIES FROM FAT	FORMULA	FAT % OF CALORIES
2 Oreo cookies	320	126	126 ÷ 320 = .393	39.3%
Lean hamburger, 4 oz (70% lean, 30% fat by weight)	380	306	306 ÷ 380 = .805	80.5%
2% Low fat milk, 8 oz	120	45	45 ÷ 120 = .375	37.5%
Whole milk, 8 oz	150	72	72 ÷ 150 = .480	48.0%

Wait a minute! How does lean hamburger get 80.5% of its calories from fat when it's 30% fat by weight?

Fat is the most high calorie food on the planet. It's more calorie-dense than the pure muscle meat in hamburger.

Millions of people are buying food with labels that confuse them. Low fat milk, low fat cheese, low fat sandwich meat. They have labels which list fat by grams, fat by percentage of weight, and fat calories. But not the percentage of calories from fat. It's so easy to get confused and think that the percentage by weight is actually the percentage of calories from fat. It's not.

Here is a photograph of an actual nutrition labels on a deli meat labeled as "Low fat":

Nutrition Facts
Serving Size 1 slice (6-1/4" x 4" x 1/16") (28 g)

Per Serving	% Daily Value*
Calories 46	
Calories from Fat 22	
Total Fat 2.4g	4%
Saturated Fat 0.8g	4%
Polyunsaturated Fat 0.2g	
Monounsaturated Fat 1.2g	
Cholesterol 16mg	5%
Sodium 365mg	15%
Potassium 80.36mg	2%
Carbohydrates 1.1g	0%
Dietary Fiber 0.4g	1%
Sugars 0g	
Protein 4.6g	

Vitamin A 0% · Vitamin C 2%

Calcium 1% · Iron 2%

Fat calories here are actually 47.8% of the item's total calories. Glancing at this label, you'd have the impression that the fat calories are just 4% of the total, because 4% jumps out at you, thanks to the layout. But, this is misleading. 4% is actually a calculation of the grams of fat calories as a percentage. of your daily calorie recommended allowance of 2,000 calories.

Confused? Me, too. Most consumers don't understand the difference between percentage-of-fat-by-weight and percentage-of-fat-by-calories. I didn't for the longest time. I would buy cheese labeled "low-fat" thinking it really was.

Producers of so-called "low-fat" meats and cheeses use this confusing fat-by-weight measurement to market foods to you that are actually quite high in fat by the American Heart Association's standards. Protect yourself from marketing folks who don't have your best interests at heart. Don't rush through the store believing only slogans used to sell packaged foods. Take a minute to calculate the fat calorie content by percentage whenever you read a nutrition label.

Think low-fat 2% milk gets 2% of the calories from fat? Think again!

Low-fat 2% milk actually gets 37.5% of its calories from fat. The 2% on the label results from calculating fat gram weight compared to overall weight of the fluid.

See how this confusion works again?

You may be buying 2% milk because you think that it's so much lower in saturated fats than whole milk. Aren't you surprised to learn that 2% milk gets nearly as many calories from fat as Oreo cookies?

Low fat foods are big business; I wish that all labels listed percentage of calories from fat so consumers wouldn't be confused.

What if the label only gives you fat grams? Here's how to convert fat grams into calories then into percentages.

Each gram of fat has 9 calories. That's true whether the fat is butter or canola oil or chicken fat. So, convert the fat grams into fat calories easily. Just multiply the grams by 9. Phones these days have calculators, so you always have a quick tool in your pocket to help out.

Here are some examples of converting fat grams to calorie percentages:

MAYONAISE: 1 TABLESPOON				
CALORIES	FAT GRAMS	CALORIES FROM FAT	FORMULA	FAT % OF CALORIES
90	10	90 (10 x 9 = 90)	90 ÷ 90 = 1.00	100%
PEANUT BUTTER, CREAMY: 1 TABLESPOON				
CALORIES	FAT GRAMS	CALORIES FROM FAT	FORMULA	FAT % OF CALORIES
100	8	72 (8 x 9 = 72)	72 ÷ 100 = .72	72%
HAM, BONELESS: 1 3 OZ SLICE				
CALORIES	FAT GRAMS	CALORIES FROM FAT	FORMULA	FAT % OF CALORIES
150	8	72 (8 x 9 = 72)	72 ÷ 150 = .48	48%

What about saturated fats?
Have they been unfairly demonized? Yes.

Americans worry a lot about the type fats we are eating because we have been taught that saturated fat raises cholesterol and causes heart disease. Starting in the 1970's, we were persuaded that removing saturated fat would lead to good health, and supermarket shelves filled up with low-fat versions of foods, like milk, yogurts and sandwich meats. Food manufacturers loved this because it gave them a reason to double their shelf space, offering low-fat versions next to regular versions. Plus, it gave them a handy sales slogan "Low fat" that consumers had been programed to respond to favorably.

This made a big impression on me as a young woman, because it was the first time in my life that eating good tasting food and danger had been directly connected. Somehow, it was hammered into my head that saturated fat was poison, and that unless I'm vigilant, my heart would become sickened. That sense of danger remains alive for many of us and it's really too bad. Every time I cook for my sons and put butter in the pan, I wonder if I'm giving them coronary disease.

But is the connection between saturated fats, raised cholesterol and heart disease actually true? Did scientists in the 1950's get it wrong? The belief that dietary fat caused heart disease spread nationally in the 20th century and dramatically influenced nutrition recommendations. Was this based on misinformation?

Apparently so. There is new, reliable news about flawed early studies and mistaken conclusions. It turns out that subsequent, multiple longterm studies have failed to find the connection. There is no empirical, scientific proof that eating dietary fat causes heart disease.

What's the result for you? Basically, you can eat animal fat without the cloud of fear that's been hanging over us for decades. I personally have started adding butter back to my diet, which is a source of delight. (Remember calories, so keep your portions moderate!)

Where can you learn more? Read *Big, Fat Surprise: Why Butter, Meat and Cheese Belong in a Healthy Diet* by Nina Teicholz. It's a breathtaking history that takes you 'behind the scenes' of how health recommendations evolve, for better or worse. She traces the history of the original studies, how nutrition policies were developed, and how the food market responded by jumping in to substitute carbohydrates and sugar for dietary fat.

CARBOHYDRATES: WHAT YOU NEED TO KNOW THE GLYCEMIC INDEX IS AN ESSENTIAL GUIDE

Discussing carbohydrates is an enormous subject. There are two chapters in this book that contain a wealth of information, *Habit #6: Avoid Added Sugars and Sweetened Drinks* and *Habit #7: Find Substitutes for Refined White Flour.* I mention these right away because Americans get many of their calories from sugar/sweeteners and baked products. These are all carbohydrates.

Carbohydrates are classified into two basic types, simple and complex. Here are the facts you need to know:

- All carbohydrates are organic molecules that contain carbon, hydrogen and oxygen.

- Our bodies can break down most carbohydrate molecules into glucose and use it for energy. (An exception is dietary fiber which is actually carbohydrate that passes through our digestive track completely intact.)

- Eating carbohydrates helps protect your body's use of protein, which is needed for cell growth and repair. Protein can also be broken down and used for energy, but then there's less for the other important bodily functions.

- **Simple carbohydrates** are sugars, which are most quickly broken down into glucose. While our cells use glucose for energy, if you're trying to lose weight, having extra glucose circulating in your blood will prevent your metabolism from drawing down on fat storage.

- Simple carbohydrates we eat include: sugar, added sweeteners and refined white flours that are stripped of all grain fiber. Eating these by themselves will cause a rise in your blood glucose levels. (Also called blood sugar levels.)

- Simple carbohydrates have little nutritional value beyond glucose, which means that you're eating calories without getting the benefits of vitamins, minerals, trace elements, protein and fiber.

- Simple carbohydrates are also found in fruits and vegetables. What makes these more desirable to eat than simple sugars by themselves is the fiber content, which slows down digestion and the rise in blood glucose levels. (The additional nutrients that whole, natural foods contain are also highly desirable. These include vitamins, minerals and trace elements.)

- **Complex carbohydrates** have molecules of more complex sugars, which require more work from your body to break down. This is a good thing because it keeps your blood sugar level more stable, longer.

- Complex carbohydrates are generally better for you to eat because they contain fiber and more nutrients. You get more benefits from the calories you've consumed.

- Eating complex carbohydrates while staying away from simple carbohydrates will help you avoid empty calories, as well as spikes and crashes in blood sugar levels.

- Complex carbohydrates also help our stomachs feel full longer.

- Complex carbohydrates are what's usually advised if you are having trouble with constipation. Fiber helps you poop regularly!

<table>
<tr><td align="center">COMMON SIMPLE CARBOHYDRATES</td></tr>
<tr><td>Soft drinks, sweetened juices, candy, white and brown sugars, honey, jam, jelly. Refined white flour and products made from it including pastries, cakes, white breads, pizza dough, cookies, crackers. Generally the word "refined" means that the ingredient has been modified to be a simple carbohydrate.</td></tr>
<tr><td align="center">COMMON COMPLEX CARBOHYDRATES</td></tr>
<tr><td>Whole grains and products made from them including oatmeal, pasta, breads. Starchy vegetables including potatoes, sweet potatoes, corn. Legumes including beans, lentils, peas. Green, red and yellow vegetables including peas, red peppers, squash.</td></tr>
<tr><td align="center">FRUITS: SIMPLE OR COMPLEX CARBOHYDRATES?</td></tr>
<tr><td>Fruits can be high in sugar, but they are usually classified as complex carbohydrates because of their fiber content.</td></tr>
</table>

The jury is <u>not</u> still out. The judgment is in and it's loud and clear. Simple carbohydrates are not as good for your health as complex carbohydrates. The solid advice for your health is to avoid them.

Unfortunately, simple carbohydrates are ubiquitous in the American food supply. There are two basic reasons for this:

- Humans love to eat sweet foods. Sweet foods sell very well. Food producers want to sell their products, so the range of foods with sweet flavors expands and expands.

- Refined white flours are easier to work with for bakers than whole grain flours. (See *Habit #7: Find Substitutes for Refined White Flour.*) Working with an easy ingredient reduces production time and increases profit. It also leads to a wider variety of possible products, which means more market presence and more sales.

Let's sum it up: Eat complex carbohydrates. Avoid simple carbohydrates.

This is not just for weight loss and weight control. It's also for your overall health. The rise of obesity, diabetes and heart disease has followed the rise in available simple carbohydrates in the American food supply. If you wish to thrive, changing your lifestyle to avoid simple carbohydrates is an excellent way to start.

THE GLYCEMIC INDEX: An essential guide for understanding carbohydrates

If you are not aware of the Glycemic Index, I recommend learning about it as an essential tool to help you manage the carbohydrate intake in your diet

Let's take a look.

In 1981, Dr. David Jenkins, and colleagues at the University of Toronto, developed clinical tests to accurately measure how quickly blood glucose rose after a person ate different foods in identical portions. This rise is the direct result of how quickly food is broken down in our digestive system. The results were ranked high to low, based on the amount of time it took to raise glucose levels, how high they went and how long they stayed elevated.

Foods with carbohydrates that raised blood glucose levels the fastest and highest were given the highest Glycemic Index ranking. Foods with carbohydrates that were slower and lower raising blood glucose levels were given the lowest Glycemic Index ranking. Then, the foods tested were grouped into High, Medium and Low categories.

The scale used is 0 – 100.

- High Glycemic rankings: 70 to 100

- Medium Glycemic rankings: 56 to 69

- Low Glycemic rankings: 0 to 55

Since slowing your digestion and avoiding blood glucose spikes is highly desirable for a weight control lifestyle, familiarizing yourself with the Glycemic Index (abbreviated to GI) make sense and is worth the effort. Basically, low GI rankings are much better food choices for you.

Foods with high GI rankings should be eaten in very limited portions, or avoided altogether.

Since the 1980s, the GI rankings have become a widespread tool to define and organize food choices. It's especially useful for diabetics who must monitor their blood glucose levels very carefully because spikes in glucose levels require an insulin response. For those of us who are not diabetics, paying attention to the Glycemic Index is one way of doing our best to not develop diabetes.

One reason the Glycemic Index is helpful today is that it's so popular and information is easy to find. This is not an obscure nutrition trend! Books, apps and free Glycemic Index charts you can download for quick reference make it simple to check on which foods to eat. You can simply follow the chart or do a deep dive into a wealth of research. As always, I encourage you to learn as much as possible. You'll find my recommended books about the Glycemic Index in the *Resource* section.

Remember, eating low on the Glycemic Index is the best way to get your carbohydrates and avoid the consequences of high blood glucose levels. The low GI carbohydrates will be complex, with fiber and offer you vitamins, minerals and trace elements.

Don't forget portion control! Just because a food is judged to be a good carbohydrate source for you, please don't gorge on it. Calories still add up.

Here is a quick overview of foods grouped by their Glycemic Index:

THE GLYCEMIC INDEX FOOD GROUPINGS		
Low GI: 0 - 55	Most green vegetables, Most fruits, Beans, Seeds and nuts, Whole grains.	Make these foods the focus of your eating: Spinach, kale, artichokes, asparagus, lettuce, zucchini Peaches, strawberries, blueberries, apricots, grapefruit Soy, lima, butter, black, kidney, lentil, kidney, chickpea Sunflower, flax, sesame, walnuts, cashews, almonds Durum wheat, oat, rice, rye, barley, spelt, millet
Medium GI: 56 - 69	Starchy vegetables, Juicy & dried fruits, Grains – not whole, Some vegetables, Breakfast cereals.	Eat these foods only in moderation: Sweet potatoes, yams, green peas, Grapes, bananas, cantalope melon, papaya, dried fruits Corn, oatmeal, Raisin Bran, Special K, whole wheat bread, white rice, whole wheat pasta, popcorn
High GI: 70 - 100	Sweet desserts of all kinds, Sweetened cereals, Sweetened drinks, Beer, Potatoes.	Avoid these foods if possible and find substitutes: Candy, chocolate, cakes, cookies, pies, cupcakes, donuts, pastries, sweetened breakfast cereals Sweetened sodas, milk shakes, watermelon, Potatoes, pumpkin Beer, cider

HABIT #6
AVOID ADDED SUGARS
& SWEETENED DRINKS

**Be aware of sugar hiding in your food,
and how it stimulates your brain's pleasure center
You can move past wanting sugar!
Alcohol: What's your best choice for weight control?**

Ten thousand years ago, the only sugar crop in the world grew on the South Pacific island of New Guinea. The native tribes there worshipped the sugar cane. In fact, they believed that the human race started when the first man made love to a sugarcane stalk. Sex and sugar. Can you imagine a more tantalizing combination for ancient humans? You know, some things haven't changed!

Today, sugar has conquered the planet. Some form is eaten in every country and Americans eat the sweetest diet in human history. We not only love the sweet taste on our tongues but chemically, sugars hijack our brain's reward center demanding that we eat more. Some form of sugar seems to be everywhere in our lives.

And yet *there is absolutely no nutritional reason you need to eat any sugar at all, in any form*: loose sugar, cooked sugar, sweet drinks or sweeteners, honey, corn syrup or any other type of sweetener.

You could survive and thrive beautifully without another drop of sugar ever crossing your lips. Some of my friends think this would be a fate worse than death, but we all agree that it's easy to eat too darn much sugar. Our ancestors could eat an occasional sweet fruit, but today, there's sugar on every corner available for us. Plus, sugars are often hidden ingredients, which makes avoiding them even more of an obstacle course, especially if we eat packaged foods without bothering to read the nutrition labels.

Sugar has an immensely strong effect on your brain and on your metabolism. Our brains are finely tuned chemical systems which are constantly hard at work, waking and sleeping, reacting to the food, drink and drugs we put in our bodies.

Having a better understanding about your food environment and how your body reacts to sugar is vital to your success with weight control.

Let's start with the basics.

Glucose, sucrose, fructose are types of sugar. They are all simple carbohydrates that digest quickly.

The reason to understand the commonly eaten sugars and their differences is because this will help you avoid what you don't need. "Sugar" is a generic word but the actual identifiers like "sucrose", "glucose", "fructose" and "lactose" are more accurate. The ending "ose" comes from the Greek and means "sweet".

- **Sucrose** is table sugar.

- **Glucose** is dietary sugar contained inside a plant or animal body.

- **Fructose** is the sugar in fruit and some vegetables like corn.

- **Lactose** is the sugar in milk products.

Because all of these forms of sugars are simple carbohydrates that digest quickly, they move out of your stomach and into your bloodstream and reach your brain really fast. Then, depending on the type of sugar, these simple carbohydrates travel around the body to different destinations.

Here's where it gets confusing: when you eat sucrose (table sugar) your body breaks down the sucrose molecules into two different sugars: glucose and fructose. So, sucrose actually ceases to exist and is used by your metabolism as glucose and fructose. Now, if you eat fructose directly, as in high fructose corn syrup, your body doesn't break it down in the same way but we'll get to that in a minute. Let's focus on glucose.

Glucose is the most common type of sugar on Earth

Glucose is one of the primary products made by plants with photosynthesis and thus is found all over the world. All cells, plant and animal, need energy to work, and glucose is the most common energy fuel.

All animals use glucose in their metabolism. In fact, inside your body, your cells are using glucose right this moment. Your brain is the biggest user, which is why the consumption of any type of sugar affects your behavior so much. Your brain is only 2% of your body weight but it uses up 20% of your daily internal energy consumption.

Normally, people don't eat glucose directly. Glucose by itself, as it turns out, doesn't taste so sweet. The sweet taste we enjoy comes from sucrose and fructose. You can buy glucose tablets and liquid, but as a raw material, it's used mostly for baking or making candy.

You can get glucose from eating plants and animal products. It's present in every one of those cells. You don't need to eat sweet foods to get the glucose you need for your body's energy.

After you absorb the glucose from whatever the source, your body doesn't leave it alone. It's joined with proteins and enzymes by your metabolism to form other chemicals you need to live, and it's also broken down into a variety of bio-molecular compounds including organic carbon. All forms of glucose are water soluble.

Not all organs are happy to receive glucose in your bloodstream. Your pancreas reacts to glucose in your blood by producing extra insulin to reduce high glucose levels. You know that insulin spiking up and down is a problem for diabetics. It's thought that the human pancreas can get worn out producing insulin spikes over time, and that's why excessive intake of sugars is a primary cause of Type 2 diabetes.

Remember: you can get all the glucose you need to thrive and live well from eating plants and meat. There is absolutely no health reason to eat any form of sugar by itself. Sweeteners are a source of pleasure, not survival.

Why do children crave sweets?

If you're the parent of young children, you are painfully aware of their constant demand for sweet food. There are two simple reasons for this:

Reason #1: Young children have undeveloped taste buds on their tongues and can't recognize all flavors. Sweet is the dominant flavor they know because taste buds sensitive to sweet develop first as we grow.

Adult tongues have between 2,000 – 4,000 taste buds that can taste salty, sour, bitter and umami (savory) as well as sweet. This is why adults appreciate complex flavors but children clamor for sweets.

Reason #2: Children's bodies are growing fast and glucose is energy. When humans lived in the wild before civilization developed, a sweet taste signaled food that was full of nutrients and safe to eat. It makes sense that our taste buds would recognize these first.

As adults, our taste buds are very individualized. Some of us prefer salty foods, as I do. One of my sons loves sour flavors and even as a teenager would eat sour candy that made me gag. Just know that if you have a preference for sweets, it's natural, especially if you were fed a lot of sugar as a child. (See *Part One: Start by Learning Why You are Unique* for information on how childhood preferences are developed and can be relearned.)

How much added sugar can you eat?
Here are recommendations.

There is no mystery to how much added sugar you need: zero. But most of us love sweetened foods and want to enjoy ourselves. The solution is portion control—knowing how much you can safely eat and still be able to control your weight.

The American Heart Association (AHA), suggests the **maximum amount** of added sugars you should eat in a day are:

- **Women:** 100 calories per day (25 grams or 6 teaspoons).

- **Men:** 150 calories per day (37.5 grams or 9 teaspoons).

Here's how to convert grams into calories: Each gram is 4 calories, so multiple your total grams by 4. (Ex: 37.5 grams x 4 calories = 150 calories per gram.)

Try to memorize that each gram of sugar is 4 calories because most packaged foods list added sugar content only by grams. You must know this conversion rate to understand what you're eating.

The women's portion of 6 teaspoons seems like a lot of sugar if you just sit down with a sugar bowl. But it's easily hidden in prepared foods. For example, one popular fat free yogurt, Yoplait's 6 oz Blueberry, has 6 ½ teaspoons or 27 grams of sugar in just one container. That's your entire day's allowance!

Reading labels is important!! This is a skill for weight control that can't be stressed enough, but labels about sugar don't make it easy for you. There may be many different types of sugars in the same food, some of which have long chemical names most non-chemists don't understand.

Your will power and self-control are affected by the sugars you eat

Added sugars sabotage your efforts at self-control. Stay away from them.

Eating too much added sugar has powerful consequences for your self-control.

Glucose enters the bloodstream and circulates to the brain, but it also goes to the pancreas, which recognizes the high glucose levels and creates extra insulin. The insulin is supposed to bond with glucose, pull it out of circulation, and bring the blood back into optimal balance.

But the plan goes haywire when too much insulin causes the glucose level to fall too low. This is what we call a "sugar crash". Your (now confused) brain knows that the glucose in your blood is out of balance so it releases the signal to "Eat! Eat! Find more glucose!" You might feel shaky and uncomfortable. And you need to eat again. Soon.

The net result of eating too much sugar is that is so much harder to control how many calories you eat and when you want to eat. It will be more difficult to make practical choices about food when you feel uncomfortable and need to raise your blood sugar quickly.

Do you crave sugary foods? Here are the real reasons why: our brain's "Reward Center" and dopamine.

Sugars are hard to resist, especially if you're in the habit of loading them into your body over the years. You may find it very difficult to stop. It's very much the same as withdrawing from a drug.

Here's why: Your brain has a strong metabolic response to glucose in your bloodstream and one of those responses is to trigger the release of dopamine. This is the same chemical that stimulates the brain with the use of heroin, cocaine, methamphetamine and marijuana. Oh, boy.

No wonder we love sweets! No wonder it's so hard to seriously cut back!

Dopamine affects your motivation and ability to make decisions. In the brain, it's a neurotransmitter that turns on the "Reward Center" which tells your conscious mind that you're feeling good. Part of your mind may feel guilty about indulging in sugary foods because you know they're not good for your health, but it's your Reward Center that makes sugars irresistible. You feel great when you eat them. You feel up! You feel energized! That's the effect of dopamine.

Properly, the Reward Center is known as the "nucleus accumbens". (Try dropping that name at a birthday party after a bite of cake. "Oooh, my nucleus accumbens is feeling soooo good! Think I'll have another slice.")

Two hormones participate in telling the Reward Center what to do: insulin and leptin. Leptin was only discovered in 1994 and is not as widely know as insulin, so don't feel badly if you haven't heard of it yet. Surprisingly, most leptin is made by your fat cells. When it's released, leptin travels in the bloodstream to tell your Reward Center that you're full and satisfied, and you want to stop eating.

Leptin suppresses the release of dopamine. But this doesn't happen when there is too much insulin in your system.

Insulin and leptin interact strongly. When you eat sugary foods, insulin spikes in your bloodstream in response to all that extra glucose and the resulting extra insulin acts as a block against your brain's ability to read the leptin message. When your brain is flooded with insulin, it can't receive the leptin message to stop releasing dopamine.

Your Reward Center continues to be dopamine stimulated.

Your craving for sugary foods has a true metabolic reason

Eating anything but very small portions of sugars throws your insulin and leptin out of balance, which then affects how much dopamine circulates in your system. Some doctors think that foods full of sugars are just as powerful as drugs and are just as addicting. (I especially recommend the book *Fat Chance: Beating the Odds Against Sugar, Processed Food, Obesity, and Disease* by Robert H. Lustig, M.D., M.S.L. You could also watch his YouTube video: *Sugar: The Bitter Truth.*)

If you can avoid eating sugary foods, your insulin, leptin and dopamine will fall back into their natural regulating levels. This is true unless you have a serious metabolic disorder. But withdrawing from sugars isn't easy for most people; don't underestimate how powerful sugar's effect is on your metabolism. The lure of keeping dopamine in your system is very strong.

What about a "sugar detox"? A small industry has sprung up to help wean people off sugar. I recommend consulting a licenses nutritionist for a plan specific to your needs. To learn more about it in the meanwhile, there are several sensible-sounding programs with easily available publications. You'll find a selection of sugar detox books in *Part Five: Resources for Learning More.* There are also specific suggestions for finding help with your cravings in *Habit #10: Control Your Food Cravings.*

Giving up sugar isn't easy but it can be done! Thousands of people have done it and you can join them. I've done it and am healthier and happier living a life with firm control on limiting added sugar!

Let's talk about fructose

Fructose is fruit sugar only found in plants, where it is often bonded to glucose. Fructose is the most water-soluble of all types of sugar, which makes it very useful for creating drinks.

Fructose is also the sweetest of all sugars, drop for drop. The human tongue is a sensitive organ and will detect fructose in a mixture before it detects sucrose.

You can see the appeal fructose has for food manufacturing companies. It's highly water soluble so it's easy to mix, is very sweet, and the flavor explodes in your mouth quickly. Throw in newish technology that inexpensively produces fructose from corn, add in government subsidies to grow millions of tons of corn and you have a winning combination for food producers! Low cost. Easy production. Satisfied customers. High profits.

Fructose is a fabulously successful ingredient in today's food supply chain—its consumption is at an all-time high and growing. The average American now eats over 69 pounds of high fructose corn syrup (HFCS) every year. That's a lot! Try to guess how many shopping bags full of breakfast cereal, bread, soda, snack bars and candy someone needs to eat to come up with 69 pounds of HFCS. My stomach hurts thinking about it!

Why too much fructose is a health hazard: Your liver turns fructose into fat.

Here's how your body deals with the fructose you eat:

- Your metabolism has limited options. Fructose won't bond to proteins and enzymes in the same useful ways as glucose does, so our bodies have a more limited range of ways that fructose can be digested and processed.

- The liver alone has exclusive enzymes to break down fructose and pull it out of circulation. Glucose can be used by every cell in your body and most especially by your brain. Not so fructose. This wasn't well known until recently.

- Fructose has the distinction of being the most lipogenic carbohydrate. "Lipogenic" means fat making.

<u>What happens is this: your liver turns fructose into fat.</u> Some fat is sent to fat cells, some is stored directly in the liver, which results in fatty liver disease. And the real fun has just begun. Metabolizing fructose increases inflammation, promotes heart disease, creates insulin resistance, helps many cancers to grow because of high insulin levels. In addition, metabolizing fructose can cause gout or create a "leaky gut" which causes more inflammation, and...get ready for this....ages your body faster because of all this inflammation.

And I haven't even said "diabetes" yet.

So, why can't we just deal with this stuff? What makes fructose such a difficult material for humans to digest when it tastes so great?

It's thought that our ancestors grew up only having occasional sweet fruits...when they were lucky to find them. Their digestive systems never had to deal with a frequent flood of fructose, so we humans never evolved to process large amounts of what was once a very rare material. Today, our food environment is so different. You can find snacks with fructose on every corner.

Fructose is everywhere in our foods because it's so darn cheap. Did it cause the American Obesity Epidemic?

A pound of high fructose corn syrup costs 13 cents at wholesale. A pound of table sugar made from beets costs 24 cents. (2005 numbers.) If one manufacturing material costs half the price of another, which would you use if you were running a factory? And, remember that HFCS is more water soluble and tastes sweeter, so it's an ideal ingredient: cheap, easy to work with, effective.

That's why there are enormous amounts of HFCS in circulation in the US food supply. In terms of production, there are now 700 calories available every day to every person just from sugars. These are calories that have absolutely no nutritional value. They are empty calories.

Is it a co-incidence that the US obesity rates started exploding in the 1980's, just when the technology to mass-produce cheap sweetener from corn became widespread? Are Americans becoming so obese because their fructose consumption is metabolized into fat or, have millions become obese just because so many more calories are available for so little money? The answers to these questions are hotly debated by nutritionists, doctors and research scientists.

One thing that everyone agrees on is that high fructose corn syrup was not widespread in the American food supply until the 1980's. I remember corn syrup in my mother's kitchen as a jar of Caro, which was only used rarely in baking. If you grew up before 1980 you just didn't eat as many calories from sugars as Americans who have grown up after 1980. I agree with those who think that the flood of HFCS starting 1980's is a real tipping point in the American diet and the Obesity Epidemic. (For an excellent overview of the rise of HFCS in our food supply, read *Fast Food Nation* by Eric Schlosser. You'll find it, along with many other books I recommend in the *Resource* section.)

Fructose disrupts your biochemical communication system. It short-circuits your brain's ability to send messages.

As we discussed before, fructose is metabolized differently than glucose. Our bodies can't digest it the same way – it won't bond to the enzymes and proteins used to break down glucose. The only way our bodies can deal with this substance is by sending it to our livers. There, specialized enzymes break down fructose into fats.

Here's what's missing when you consume fructose: your brain doesn't receive the biochemical signal that your blood sugar is high so it can respond. No "stop being hungry" messages are sent. No "I'm full now" messages are sent. When you eat fructose, your brain never registers that it has enough.

Haven't you ever wondered how people could possibly drink those enormous sodas without wanting to throw up? Sure, there's volume pressure in the stomach or the need to pee, but if soda or juice is sweetened by high-fructose corn syrup you can drink more because there is no metabolic message to stop. The drinking can go on and on, and when that fructose gets to your liver, it's converted to fat. Directly.

My strong recommendation is to avoid eating or drinking anything with high fructose corn syrup

Take care of yourself while the scientists debate how dangerous high fructose corn syrup is for public health. It's clear enough that HFCS doesn't provide anything you need for your health. Humans survived nicely without it until the 1980's.

These are the basic actions you need to take to protect yourself from high fructose corn syrup:

- Read the labels if you're buying something in a package or a bottle and, if it contains HFCS, put it back on the shelf. Tell your grocer that you want foods that are healthy and not full of added sweeteners.

- Avoid junk foods and fast foods whenever possible.

- Don't drink sodas or sweetened fruit juices. Americans get 20% of their calories from sodas and sweetened drinks! Be smart and learn to give up sweetened sodas.

What about fruit? Isn't that fructose?

Fruit eaten whole is not a problem. Yes, it's sweet and contains small amounts of fructose, but eating a piece of fruit will give you fiber, antioxidants, vitamins and minerals. These are all very good for you.

Eat the fruit.

What about honey, maple syrup, molasses and agave syrup?

Only a very small percentage of sweeteners consumed by most Americans are from bees and trees. Molasses is made from sugar cane, grapes or sugar beets and is a common ingredient in baking, but most molasses produced in the world today is used to make rum. It's also used as an ingredient in cattle feed.

All four of these naturally sweet products contain traces of vitamins and minerals. Historically, Blackstrap molasses was an important source of calcium, potassium, iron and magnesium.

Agave syrup is a recent addition to grocery store shelves. It comes from the blue agave cactus (which also gives us tequila) and is being marketed as a healthy sweetener based on dubious claims as a low-glycemic food. In actuality, agave syrup contains high amounts of fructose and so should be treated with the same care you would use with high fructose corn syrup.

In my own kitchen, I keep all four of these sweeteners as flavor additives, especially for breakfast foods. But, I use them sparingly, like a treat. Try to remember that before you drown your pancakes in maple syrup. Instead, use the same trick of dipping your fork that is so popular for salad dressings: put the maple syrup in a portion-control small bowl. Dip your fork in the syrup before picking up a bite of pancake. You'll get the sweet taste. This works!

A word about lactose

Lactose is the sugar in milk products and is generally not a concern when we talk about eating too much sugar. Sure, you can gorge on cheese, which has lactose, but the primary concern with cheese is the calories from fat. And, you don't hear complaints about children drinking supersized cups of milk.

I became lactose intolerant in my late twenties. Cheese and my beloved café lattes gave me horrible stomach aches because my body stopped producing lactase, the digestive enzyme needed to break down lactose. Dairy Aid lactose pills were hard to find back then, so I reluctantly gave up eating most milk products. Yes, that means that I haven't had a slice of pizza in years. I do miss it very, very much. But, so many years later, life without cheese is filled with many other pleasures. And, it's obvious how many calories I'm saving.

Today, you can buy lactose digestive enzyme pills in any drug store, and I carry a bottle of them in my purse. This is so when I'm out to lunch or dinner with friends and cheese is served, I don't have to make a fuss. I discretely chew a few Dairy Aid pills and eat what's put in front of me.

For those of you who are also lactose intolerant, perhaps, like me, you see this as a blessing for weight control.

A note about yogurt: there are two reasons why lactose intolerant people can often eat Greek yogurt. First: the processing removes much of the milk's whey and its lactose. And second: yogurt contains live active cultures, (also called probiotics), help break down the lactose that remains.

Greek yogurt, whole milk, especially plain, unflavored and unsweetened, is good food, high in protein with 11 grams per cup. The lactose adds up to 9 grams of sugar per cup, or 36 sugar calories. A cup of whole milk, plain Greek yogurt only has 200 calories and makes a great snack or dessert.

Why food manufacturers love added sugars and use them in so many products

You'd expect to find sweeteners in candy and sweet breakfast cereal, but what about your hamburger bun, French fries, or spaghetti sauce? That "healthy" non-fat yogurt has as much sweetener as a candy bar!

Here are three reasons why added sugars are such a valued ingredient for food manufacturers:

- Sugar extends the shelf-life of packaged foods. It acts like a preservative while improving flavor. Sugar is particularly useful in bread from large bakeries because it camouflages the taste of dough conditioners and preservatives.

- Government subsidies make high fructose corn syrup a very inexpensive ingredient. In a business environment where delivering profits is key, using cheap ingredients holds down costs and boosts profits. You could argue that your tax dollars are helping to make you fat and give you diabetes.

- Being scared of high-fat foods gave manufacturers the opportunity to increase flavor with sweeteners. We learned to be scared of high-fat diets when they were blamed for heart disease in the 1970's. Food manufacturers responded with marketing an explosion of low-fat packaged foods that got their flavor from sweeteners. "Low-fat" or "non-fat" is a claim that continues to sell products packed with sweeteners because most people don't read the ingredients label— they just scan the marketing copy on the front of the box and ignore the high sugar content.

HOW TO AVOID ADDED SUGARS: HERE'S WHAT YOU NEED TO DO

The place to start is accepting that there is absolutely no nutritional reason you need to eat any form of added sugar, cooked sugar, sweet drinks or sweeteners of any kind. We eat sweeteners for pleasure only. You can get all the glucose your body needs from vegetables, legumes, grains and meat.

Follow these tips to reduce the amount of added sugars in your diet.

20 TIPS TO AVOID ADDED SUGARS	
Tip #1	Don't skip meals. When you are very hungry, it's easier to overeat. Remember that all sugars are simple carbohydrates and metabolize very fast. That's why we reach for them when we're uncomfortably hungry.
Tip #2	Snacking on foods rich in fiber is helpful. (Apples, vegetables, whole grains.) Your blood glucose will stay stable, and you won't feel desperate to reach for a sugary treat.
Tip #3	Plan ahead to have healthy snacks available. Take a trip down the fruit aisle or your supermarket. At your local coffee shop, buy an apple, orange or banana for a snack later in the day.
Tip #4	Visuals matter. Don't leave sweetened food sitting around. Keep temptation off your kitchen counters, your desk and out of your refrigerator. Keep a fruit bowl with fruit like apples out in a central, easily-seen place in your kitchen.
Tip #5	If you are at work and can't avoid seeing donuts or other sweets, chew a piece of sugarless gum and try to turn away.
Tip #6	Limit candy, baked goods and sweet desserts to pre-arranged small portions arranged carefully on a plate and don't give yourself more than three mouthfuls. See Habit #4: Learn and Practice Portion Control to tips on how to be successful limiting yourself.
Tip #7	Never eat out of wrappers.
Tip #8	Don't tempt yourself by going into bakeries or looking at candy displays. Out of sight, out of mind.
Tip #9	Have water, unsweetened coffee or tea always available to help control the urge to put something in your mouth. Carry sugarless gum with you all the time.
Tip #10	Juice is not your friend. Eat a piece of whole fruit instead. Commercially processed "juice" may be mostly sugar water. Read the label to know what's inside the bottle. You'd be better off learning to drink water and avoid juice.
Tip #11	Avoid processed foods whenever possible. Buy whole foods instead.
Tip #12	If you must eat at a fast food place, don't order soda with sugar and never order milkshakes. Water and diet sodas are a better choice.
Tip #13	Never buy sweetened sodas from a vending machine.

Tip #14	Read the nutrition labels when you buy packaged foods. Select for brands that have fewer grams of sugars per portion. 1 gram = 4 calories.
Tip #15	Remember your sugar limits for good health, according to the American Heart Association. For women: 100 calories = 25 grams or 6 teaspoons. For men: 150 calories per day = 37 ½ grams or 9 teaspoons.
Tip #16	Get enough sleep. This is very important! Sleep and being well-rested is critical for weight control. Being sleep deprived affects your judgment. See Habit #1: Get Enough Sleep.
Tip #17	Reduce alcohol to one drink per day. Wine and beer are nothing but sugars and drinking impairs your judgment.
Tip #18	Make a list of sugary foods to severely limit or avoid entirely and post it where you will see it frequently. My list includes: sodas, juices and any sweetened drinks, beer, wine, table sugar, brown sugar, molasses, any yogurt with sweetener, sweet bakery products and bread with sweeteners (read the label!), maple syrup, jams and jellies with sweetener, peanut butter with sweeteners, beer, wine, ice cream and sweet frozen desserts.
Tip #19	Take control of your power as the consumer! Stop being manipulated by advertisements selling you sweetened products. Remember that sweeteners are inexpensive ingredients so the more you buy, the food companies want to make profits. It's impossible to avoid food advertisements, but you can learn to see them for what they are: just sales tools to get you to buy products with a high profit margin. Instead, believe that you have power as a consumer to influence the food market. Invest your money towards your health, not a company's bottom line. Buy food without added sweeteners

ALCOHOL:
WINE, BEER, DISTILLED SPIRITS
What's your best choice for weight control?

Every civilization around the world has some form of alcoholic drink. Whether it's from fermented grapes (wine), fermented grains (beer), distilled from potatoes or coconut palms (vodka and kava), wherever humans have settled, they have made it a priority to convert plants into an alcoholic drink.

Some types of alcohol have surprising nutrients. Guinness dark beer actually contains fiber! (3.2 grams per 8 ounces.) Wine gets the most health and nutrition attention, because red wines contain bioflavonoids and polyphenols (strong antioxidants) which are seen as beneficial for cardiovascular health. In fact, red wine is now extolled as helping to prevent heart disease. It's a complicated claim because of all the variables and risk factors, but studies are consistently showing that drinking moderately (one drink per day) is reducing heart attacks across populations. And whether it's wine, beer or brandy doesn't seem to matter. (See *Eat, Drink and Be Healthy: The Harvard Medical School Guide to Healthy Eating* by Walter Willet, MD, in *Part Five: Resources for Learning More*.)

One thing is clear: the health benefits of drinking alcohol are NOT being recommended as a reason for people to start drinking.

Where I live, drinking is a pervasive social activity. We live near the Napa Valley, enjoy the friendships of wine makers and have done countless tours of wineries and vineyards. I personally enjoy the wine country lifestyle very much. Wine is served at nearly every social gathering, especially after 5:00 pm. Most of my friends drink. One of my sons is an artisan distiller in San Francisco, the foodie and cocktail capital of the nation.

And….I don't drink.

I stopped drinking in my 30's when I was pregnant and never started again. I just didn't feel good after drinking any kind of wine, beer or spirits, and believe me, I tried to find a drink I could enjoy. Alcohol just doesn't work with my metabolism, and after a year or so of trying, I gave up and became everyone's designated driver.

Sometimes I'd love to join my friends, but then I remember that I save calories every day by not drinking. Plus, my judgment isn't affected by alcohol. If I'm at a celebration, especially one with lots of desserts and temptations, drinking hasn't altered my self-control.

Overall, I believe that not drinking has been a major benefit to my weight control efforts. But, it's not a choice for everyone.

To drink or not to drink, for weight control?

If you drink, how can you manage your alcohol consumption for optimal weight control? Start by familiarizing yourself with the carbohydrates and calories.

Alcoholic drinks are simple carbohydrates that will be rapidly broken down by your digestive system. We discussed simple and complex carbohydrates (*Habit #5: Know What's in Your Food*) and how it's a stronger choice for weight control to stick with complex carbs and avoid foods with simple carbs.

This is true for alcoholic drinks as well. As simple carbohydrates, the most wise choice is to limit or avoid them for optimal weight loss and weight control.

All forms of alcohol have calories that add up fast. If you drink, please consider your alcohol calories as empty calories. You may remember the recommendation to restrict yourself to 160 empty calories per day. That's one glass of wine or beer.

Here are the average calorie counts for popular alcoholic drinks:

DRINK	PORTION	CALORIES*
Beer (average)	8 oz	153
Beer (dark)	8 oz	162
Beer (light)	8 oz	103
Red wine	5 oz	125
White wine	5 oz	121
Sweet wine (sherry)	3.5 oz	165
Distilled spirits (gin, vodka, whiskey, tequila)	1.5 oz	97

Calories will vary by brand. Source: National Institute of Health

There is no reliable way to list calories from cocktails as the mixes vary so wildly in ingredients and portion size. Just be aware that, since cocktails can be very strong, and contain sweet juices or syrups, they generally tend to be very caloric.

The National Institute of Health has a useful guide called *Rethinking Drinking: Alcohol and Your Health*. They recommend that to lose weight, you stop or limit your drinking. To learn more, go to: *http:// rethinkingdrinking.niaa.nih.gov*

All of that said, responsible drinking is part of our 21st century lifestyle. If you can manage your daily calorie total to include a glass or wine or beer, I haven't found any general medical advice that recommends complete abstinence. Moderation, as always, is the secret to enjoying so many of life's pleasures.

HABIT #7
FIND SUBSTITUTES FOR
REFINED WHITE FLOUR

It's a simple carbohydrate that metabolizes very fast with little nutrition to offer you.
The many benefits of eating whole grains instead.

If the saga of the American diet were written as a novel, there would be four villains:

- Refined white flour, sugar, high-fructose corn syrup and excess dietary fats. Many doctors would want to add a fifth villain: excess salt.

If the novel were one of love and loss, the story would be that the villains have won. We love to eat them and that love is causing the loss of our health.

This chapter is about the villain that is the hardest to avoid: refined white flour. Most of us are eating this every day, from pancakes to hamburger buns to snack chips to the crusty and beautiful sourdough baguettes we love in San Francisco.

If you are avoiding gluten, you have a running start at reading labels and paying attention to the grain content in your food. You are fortunate because probably you are already familiar with alternatives to wheat like millet, quinoa and farro and how to shop for them. This is high-value information.

Refined white flour from wheat has conquered the American bread basket. The entire supply chain is well-established, well-funded and well-served by corporations with billions of dollars invested to see that you continue to consume as much refined white flour as possible. In fact, your tax dollars are supporting the flood of refined white flour in the form of subsidies to wheat farmers.

Americans now get 20% of their average daily calories from foods made from refined white wheat flour. You can't avoid seeing it—the distribution of foods made from white flour is too universal. But...once you know what it does to your body and your health, will you be able to resist? The question is *can you avoid putting white flour in your mouth and will you be willing to make the effort to find alternatives?*

What is a whole grain? What's missing in white flour?

Whole grain is the entire seed of a grain plant (wheat, oat, barley, rice, millet, etc.) that has all of its original parts in the same proportions that it had in nature. It may be ground up into flour but nothing has been removed by processing.

Seeds for grains are most often called "kernels". Like all seeds, they contain three basic parts which are needed to germinate a new plant.

All three basic parts must be present in whole grain products:

PART OF THE ORIGINAL GRAIN KERNEL	WHAT IT IS	WHAT HAPPENS IN REFINED WHITE FLOUR
Bran	The outside layer of the grain. The coating of the seed.	Removed. It has a bitter taste so removing makes flour taste sweeter. Often used for animal feed.
Germ	The embryo. The fertile, reproductive part of the grain	Removed. Often used for animal feed.
Endosperm	The largest part of the grain, mostly starch, inside the bran	The starchy part that's ground up to create flour, which is white because other seed parts have been removed.

The bran and germ are the most important, nutritious part of the seed. They are rich in protein and fiber and also contains vitamins such as Vitamin E, folic acid, B vitamins (Niacin, Thiamin and B6) and minerals (including iron, magnesium, selenium and zinc).

In contrast, the endosperm is mostly starch, simple carbohydrates and contains little in the way of other nutrients. When you eat flour made from ground endosperm (all refined flours) you get very little besides calories.

Refined white flour contains only the endosperm

Refined white flour has been stripped of the grain's valuable parts—the bran and germ with their fiber and proteins have been removed. This process creates flour that is easy to work with and is pleasant pale color, which is especially useful for cakes and pastries. As our food supply became more industrialized, creating flour that was standardized really helped bakers make more products for less money. But, while this is fine for the producers' profit margin, it left the buying public with baked food stripped of vital nutrients. That's why you see the word "Fortified" on many bread labels. Producers are adding vitamins and minerals back into the blanched, stripped flour.

Flour wasn't always so stripped and devoid of nutrients. Before modern equipment, the entire grain kernel was ground up. The development of modern machinery, along with chemicals to extend flour's shelf life, and shorten baking time, have been godsends for industrial-scale food producers. But, along the way, essential nutrients have been stripped out.

What makes refined white flour so bad for your health?

The powder left after the nutrient-rich parts of the grain have been removed is primarily starch. This kind of starch is made from multiple chains of glucose molecules. It lacks fiber, vitamins, and minerals and has very little protein. Refined white flour as produced today does only one thing: deliver calories in an easily digestible form that can quickly be broken down in glucose, the energy source used by every living cell.

Originally, the wheat grain would have used its starch to make energy to grow roots, shoots and leaves for the wheat plant. The grain is, after all, a seed. The starch it held inside was fuel until its roots could pick up nutrients from the soil.

So, really, nature intended wheat starch to be temporary source of energy, just enough fuel for the plant to get started and find a more permanent supply for what it needs to grow and thrive.

You have to marvel at the irony that we, the planet's most evolved species, have taken a plant's temporary fuel and turned it into one of our primary foods—food that millions of people are consuming in vast quantities. It's a dead-end for us. As wheat flour is processed today, it cannot deliver the nutrients our bodies need to thrive. And...we can't grow roots.

Before modern, industrial processing of grains, common flour was much more nutritious because it contained all parts of the grain. Today, you need to read labels and hunt for whole grain flours. It's sad that a lot of what are called "multi-grained" products are, in reality, probably refined wheat flour with a sprinkling of other grains and coloring to make them look brown.

WHAT HAPPENS WHEN YOU EAT THE SIMPLE CARBOHYDRATES IN REFINED WHITE FLOUR?

So, what happens when we eat refined white flour?

It delivers empty calories and possibly endangers our body's longterm ability to process glucose. Refined white flour is highly processed material and should be avoided whenever possible.

Here's why:

You chew the white bread, swallow, and your digestive system gets to work quickly breaking it down into what it's made of: glucose. Starch is actually multiple glucose chains that need to be broken down into single glucose molecules. There is no fiber to slow down the process so glucose floods into your bloodstream very rapidly. Your pancreas responds by making extra insulin to force the glucose into your muscles and brain.

Your metabolism is put into overdrive. The bad news is that if your muscles are already oversaturated or insulin resistant, that glucose is stored as fat. Plus, insulin succeeds in cleaning up your blood glucose so efficiently that it drops too low and you feel hungry again. Quickly.

This is a cycle that you should know well by now. Simply put: Glucose in = insulin spike up.

The hardest part for a lot of people is learning which foods that look like normal, nutritious things to eat—like tasty breads—are actually simple carbohydrates which should be avoided. Most of us know by now that candy gives you a sugar rush followed by a sugar crash. But, most of us are not aware that the innocent looking hamburger bun, made with refined white flour, is really the first-cousin to candy. Just like candy, that white bread is metabolized as the simple carbohydrate it really is.

Remember: when you eat refined white flour, it's not just that you are depriving your body of the nutrients it needs with those empty calories, but you are actively endangering your health by forcing your system to process excessive glucose without fiber.

Are you older? That's another reason to avoid refined white flour/simple carbohydrates

Most people become more insulin resistant as they get older and become less active. Plus, our muscle and fat cells grow less sensitive to insulin as we age so more of the glucose we're eating gets stored as fat. You could be eating the same amount but your aging body is able to process less of it. This is why it is so easy to gain weight when we're older. Personally, as an older woman, I hate this!

What's the solution? Eat fewer simple carbohydrates! Eat less white bread!

Take a bite of the birthday cake instead of having the whole piece. Share the cookie. Order your sandwiches with wraps instead of bread. Switch over to whole grain pastas and crackers. If you bake, find whole grain flour or, if your recipes absolutely need white flour, enjoy giving away your pies and cakes. Limit eating pancakes or waffles to small portions on special occasions. Don't even think about the breadbasket on the restaurant table.

It really works. The more you can avoid refined white flour, the more successful you will be at controlling your weight.

Common refined white flour products to avoid

It's not easy sidestepping refined white flour. The stuff is simply everywhere you find food being offered. From waffles to French bread, most white flour used by food producers is just the norm in today's American food supply.

Question the baked products you see and, whenever possible, read the labels looking for the words "whole grains". If you don't see these two words, assume that you are being offered a product made from refined white flour. Even if the label says "whole wheat", this is not a whole grain product. If you are at a restaurant or a friend's house, of course you won't be able to read the labels. You can probably assume that the flour used to prepare or bake the food is not whole grain. Try to eat sparingly. Treat the refined white flour products like cake. Whether it's a warm loaf of banana bread or a pancake, chances are it's made from refined white flour and will be metabolized very quickly, which is not desirable for weight control

Avoid these common products made from refined white flour:

- Hamburger and hot dog buns
- Bread baskets at restaurants
- Bread sticks
- White sandwich bread
- Pancakes and waffles
- Many breakfast cereals
- Cookies
- Cake
- Pastries
- Pizza dough
- Crackers

Don't despair. Avoid refined white flour gets easier with time and practice. You will figure out how to do this. It took me a while, and the hardest part was finding another way to eat a sandwich. Whole grain tortilla wraps, lettuce wraps, rice cakes are all useful for those of us who want to hold our lunches in our hands.

And, of course, consumer demand makes a difference. Ask your grocer for whole grain products! If you bake at home, ask for whole grain flours. When you eat at a restaurant, ask if they have whole grain products. Consumer demand can drive the market. Let your wishes be known!

THE FIBER IN WHOLE GRAINS IS GOOD TO EAT. HERE'S WHY.

Fiber in whole grains is mostly not digestible by humans, so it passes through our systems intact. In the stomach, while stomach acids break down foods and churn them into a fluid, the fiber creates a net-like structure that acts to slow down how fast any material moves through your stomach and intestines. This is a rather disgusting image, but it is a very good thing for your metabolism.

Because fiber slows down your digestion, your system has the time it needs to absorb glucose and any nutrients. If you don't have fiber and the food is sweetened or converts to glucose very quickly, your system is just flooded with glucose. This causes an insulin spike and a cascade of metabolically unhealthy reactions.

Without fiber, there is nothing for your digestive system to hang on to. The refined flour used in most breads, buns, chips and cakes is converted into a slurry that your digestive enzymes can break down very quickly. That very beautiful cupcake becomes an intestinal puddle in record time.

It's all about timing. Your comfort and your health depend on you not pouring more simple carbohydrates into your system than it can absorb at one time. Slow down your digestion with fiber!

Fiber means fewer calories per mouthful

Fiber takes up physical room, so for every bite of food with fiber, a portion of what you're chewing will be calorie free since it can't be digested and absorbed. Fiber is the friend of every eater who loves to chew and craves lots of mouth action but wants to reduce calories.

When foods are high in fiber, you are eating fewer calories in every mouthful. For weight control, this is a really important thing to know. If you actively seek out foods that are high fiber, you can simply eat more of them for the same calorie load as higher calorie, low fiber food.

Here are some examples:

- 1 tbsp of sugar = 48 calories

- 1 tbsp of oatmeal = 10 calories

- 1 tbsp of cheese = 55 calories

- 1 tbsp of apple = 15 calories

- 1 tbsp of olive oil = 120 calories

- 1 tbsp of cooked spinach = 6 calories

One way to look at high fiber foods is to consider calorie density. Foods that are calorie dense generally have very little fiber. Foods that are not calories dense, are usually rich in fiber and often water, also. For a detailed discussion about calorie density, please see *Habit #5: Know What's in Your Food Before You Put It in Your Mouth.*

High fiber foods help you feel full. For those of us who don't feel satisfied until there's a pressured, full feeling in our tummies (that would be me!), eating fiber is an important tool to know about.

Fiber only comes from plants

There is no fiber in animal products. If you eat a lot of cheese, yogurt or meat, you will get zero fiber from them.

Fiber is only found in foods that come from plants, including fruits, vegetables, whole grains, legumes, nuts and seeds.

Consider adding as many vegetables to your meals as possible to get more fiber. Use any way to add vegetables to your meat dishes. Be clever and committed to add vegetables! Good examples are broiled chicken on a Cesar salad instead of chicken by itself, or Chinese stir-fries that use small pieces of meat with vegetables. That tomato slice on your Jumbo

Jack is not enough to make a difference, because the hamburger and refined white flour bun have no fiber whatsoever.

Beans are a great source of fiber. My favorites are lentils which are easy to find and delicious to eat. If you can eat a lentil dish instead of white flour pasta, you will be making a wise weight control decision.

SPIRALIZING: A NEW, HELPFUL COOKING FAD

Maybe you've seen it on YouTube or on TV cooking shows. There's a new tool for our kitchens, the spiralizer, and I think it's terrific.

You put a vegetable or firm fruit into a spiralizer, twist, and the blades slice through to create a continuous ribbon. You can make vegetable pasta from zucchini or parsnips, spiralize sweet potatoes for flexible strands that will cook quickly. Boil, pan fry, bake or eat raw. Spiralizing your vegetables is an easy and fun way to put more fiber in your diet.

And, you can make a delicious substitute for pasta. Most pasta is made from refined white flour, and whole grain pasta is hard to find. If you love pasta and don't want to give it up, consider learning about spiralizing vegetables to make healthy fettuccini, spaghetti and linguini. The better spiralizers come with a selection of blades for different sized cuts.

You can find a recommended cookbook for spiralizing in the *Resource* section at the end of this book.

In the meantime, go to YouTube and search for "spiralizing". If you have kids, this is a fun and exciting way to get them into cooking.

THE GLYCEMIC INDEX AND WHOLE GRAIN FOODS

The Glycemic Index (GI) is an important reference to know about. (We also discuss it in *Habit #5: Know What's In Your Food Before You Put It In Your Mouth.*) In the Glycemic Index, foods are ranked by how fast the human digestive system breaks down carbohydrates into glucose molecules and absorbs them. A low Glycemic Index means that the foods are absorbed slowly. This is good. Conversely, a high Glycemic Index means that the glucose in the food is absorbed quickly. Not good. The scale goes from 0 to 100, with 100 being pure glucose.

Unsurprisingly, whole grain foods with fiber have a lower GI ranking.

Here's a quick comparison:

- White bread made from refined wheat flour: 80 average GI rank

- Whole wheat bread made from whole grain flour: 50 average GI rank

Every guide to the Glycemic Index that I've ever seen advises choosing foods that are made with whole grains because their GI ranks are lower. Breads, pasta and breakfast cereals made from whole grains digest more slowly than those made from refined white flours.

Processed foods generally have a high Glycemic Index ranking. You can simplify your life by just avoiding processed foods with added sugars and refined white flours. Focus on the following foods, which have the lowest GI rankings.

- Whole grains
- Vegetables
- Fruits
- Fish
- Lean meats
- Low-fat dairy

See the *Resource* section for recommendations on where to learn more about the Glycemic Index.

A WORD ABOUT GLUTEN-FREE

If you have Celiac Disease or are avoiding gluten, you are very experienced by now at reading labels. Just follow the same healthy guidelines choosing whole grains. You are probably already enjoying the following grains which are gluten-free: amaranth, buckwheat, corn, millet, oats, quinoa, rice, sorghum and wild rice.

I personally don't follow a gluten-free diet because I think the science is inconclusive that gluten itself is the culprit for so many of our modern day health woes. I do have genuine Celiac Disease sufferers in my family who will wind up in the hospital if they eat gluten, so I don't doubt the dangers that gluten poses for people with dangerous physical reactions. But, in my opinion, there is too much fad excitement associated with selling gluten-free products to consumers who are poorly informed. To the best of my knowledge, our metabolic reaction to excessive carbohydrates from the dominance of refined white flour in our food supply is already a health hazard.

But…all the publicity about gluten has a positive effect: Shoppers are becoming more aware of the ingredients in their food and caring passionately about what they eat for health. And, if the result is eating less refined white flour, that's a good thing.

AVOIDING REFINED WHITE FLOUR GETS EASIER WITH TIME AND PRACTICE

Eventually, you will find products made from refined white flour somewhat repulsive and feel uneasy about eating them. In this age of pastries and donuts, I understand that this sounds like a fantasy, but truly, you can retrain your tastes over time.

If I'm a guest in somebody's house for dinner, I don't make a fuss and just eat what they serve me. But, I rarely buy refined white flour products to serve in my own home except for special occasion cakes. For those of you who love sour dough bread and wonderful pastas, make them an occasional treat.

I do make sure that my kitchen is stocked with whole grain products. I like foods that crunch so boxes of *Mary's Gone Crackers* whole grain crackers are a basic at my house. (Buy them at Costco or Whole Foods.) Tortillas are inexpensive and easy to find. They make quick and easy sandwiches. It's a little tougher to find whole grain pastas but, hopefully, there is a health food store near you. Pasta packages will keep for months so one trip can cover many meals.

For whole grain flour, I recommend Bob's Red Mill, King Arthur Flour and Arrowhead Mills.

Beware of deceptive packaging! Labels are confusing. Sometimes deliberately.

Food manufacturers want to sell products. They have warehouses full of materials that cannot be converted into cash until stores put the products on their shelves and you put the products into your shopping cart. It's all about the money.

I'm not a nutritionist, but I did run a manufacturing company for over thirty years and worked with over 16,000 retailers in the US, including many Fortune 500 companies. The pressure to have products fly off the shelves was relentless. Millions of dollars are spent to study what makes people buy one product over another. Never doubt for a moment that everything possible will be done to convince you to reach for that box, including product fraud.

One thing that packaging designers have always known is that most people only read the big print and don't bother with the details. And nutritionists know that most Americans don't understand the health benefits or risks to what they are eating.

In one survey, 73% of shoppers thought that "wheat flour" was the same as "whole grain flour" because the words sounded healthy.

Most commercial "whole wheat" breads started as refined white flour with additives. Many are loaded with high fructose corn syrup and other sweeteners because the bitter and chemical tastes of preservatives need to be covered. Molasses adds a brown color. Flecks of wheat bran and cracked wheat further disguise the white flour by adding cosmetic texture.

To make matters worse, a food manufacturer might use 5% whole grain flour mixed with 95% refined white flour and still claim on the box that the product is "whole grain". "Multi-grain" is even more difficult to decipher because any of the grains used are probably not whole at all.

It's sad but true that our own Food and Drug Administration (FDA) only requires whole grain to be the first ingredient on the label for breads and cereals. That means that sweetened breakfast cereals can have whole grain slightly outnumber other ingredients by weight (easy to do if you add 30 ingredients to the mix) and, legally, the packaging can claim it's a whole grain product, when, in fact, it's mostly junk. Watch out for deceptive claims!

To control your weight for the rest of your life, pay attention to ingredients. Read the small print!

Don't be gullible and buy food based on the packaging. Be smart. Don't be seduced by the word "whole". Sure, it's firmly associated in our minds with good health, both for our bodies and for the earth, but on a package, it means nothing. It's only a marketing buzz word.

I walked through the packaged bread, cereal and cracker aisles at my local Safeway supermarket recently and counted 46 products with the word "whole" on their packaging. It's worth spending five minutes in a supermarket aisle just looking at the packaging and thinking about how you're being told to buy products.

Speaking as a mother and someone with decades of product design experience, it's disheartening to see so many claims that are misleading and downright deceptive. I'm appalled that other product and packaging designers took money to do this kind of unethical work. It's like crossing over to the Dark Side.

CHOOSE THE HEALTHIEST FOOD YOU CAN AFFORD

Money makes a difference.

When I was working and had a nice paycheck, I signed up for weekly deliveries of farm-fresh produce, right to my door. I could afford the best cuts of organic meat, wild Alaska salmon, good cheeses and $7 boxes of handcrafted crackers at the local boutique food markets San Francisco area is so famous for. It was easy to eat beautiful, healthy food because I could afford it.

Now, I'm retired and my spending is much more limited. The irony is that I have more time to go shopping but I have less money.

How much money you have available is a BIG factor in what you choose to eat. My story is common—many Americans have less money to spend now for a variety of reasons. Our prolonged recession, the addition of another child in the family, other expenses that have risen and have eaten into your wallet are just a few reasons. We can't fool ourselves and ignore that money matters. Education about healthy food choices will not solve all our dietary problems. What you can afford to spend will have a big impact on what goes into your mouth.

Fast food outlets like MacDonald's and Burger King have a primary advantage if your spending is limited: you get a lot of calories for each dollar. If you're feeding a hungry family, it can be hard to overcome the appeal of how far your $20 can go towards filling their bellies.

And….if you're working your brains out holding two jobs, how can you be expected to shop around looking for the perfect whole grain bread?

Are you facing a situation like this? Don't give up! There are strategies that will help you control your weight and avoid refined white flour. And never forget that you have the power of a consumer. As more people become aware of the dangers of processed food and demand healthier choices, retailers will respond.

20 TIPS TO AVOID REFINED WHITE FLOUR	
Tip #1	Order your sandwiches with wraps instead of bread.
Tip #2	Don't eat the bread at restaurants before the meal.
Tip #3	Substitute nuts or salted fresh vegetables for chips and pretzels when you want crunch and salt. Be pro-active! Don't wait for the crunch and salt yearning to hit you. Make sure that you have a steady stream of crunchy vegetables available throughout the day.
Tip #4	Read all labels for breads and baked products.
Tip #5	Beware of any product that claims to be "enriched". That means the nutrition was stripped out during processing and government mandated additives were put back in. Buy whole foods instead of processed foods.
Tip #6	White toast is your silent enemy. Eat whole grain crackers instead of white toast.
Tip #7	Know that processed "wheat flour" is nutritionally the same as "white flour".
Tip #8	Be willing to try new foods, especially grains and legumes.
Tip #9	Practice portion control with cakes, cookies and pies. (Yes, this is a challenge if you love to bake and eat pastries!)

Tip #10	Stock up on whole grain pasta if you cook pasta at home.
Tip #11	Don't buy junk food snacks. Really. Just don't unless you want to sabotage your weight control efforts.
Tip #12	Bring your lunch to work and make sure you're prepared to get through the day with healthy choices.
Tip #13	If you really have no choice but a fast food restaurant, order the salad option. Add grilled chicken if you eat meat but throw out the salad dressing packet.
Tip #14	Cook a large pot of whole grain once a week and use it for multiple meals.
Tip #15	Ask the manager at your local supermarket to stock more whole grain options.
Tip #16	Try stacking your food on the plate, like fancy restaurants do. Put whole grains on the bottom, then arrange vegetables, meats, condiments on top. Vertical food is attractive to eat!
Tip #17	Find the health food store or farmer's market nearest to your home. Buy a loaf of whole grain bread there and try it out. You can freeze bread easily so it will keep longer. Thaw the slices you need in a toaster. This will help you adjust to lowered bread consumption without the bread spoiling.
Tip #18	Identify reputable brands of bread, cereal and crackers and give them your business. This means not buying products with deceptive health claims on their packaging. Read the ingredients!
Tip #19	Continue to learn about nutrition. Be on the lookout for articles, TV shows, books that will help you know more.
Tip #20	Try an experiment: go breadless for a week. Be creative about substitutes. (Use wraps, lettuce leaves, whole grain crackers.) When you start eating bread again, be very careful about choosing only whole grain products.

Eating well at home is less expensive than eating out but requires time and planning ahead

We all know that buying food in bulk is a lot less expensive. Foods that keep for a long time, like beans and dry whole grains are good choices to keep in the house. You can save a considerable amount of money if you are willing to buy dry foods in bulk, then take the time to prepare them.

If buying in bulk is too much for you, and you have a Trader Joe's nearby, take a look at their wide selection of whole grains and try something new in smaller portions.

I usually focus on one whole grain for the week (like millet, brown rice, farro or quinoa) and start by cooking a large potful flavored with broth or vegetables. I use a scoop of this grain as the base for most dinners that week, adding vegetables, proteins and combining leftovers as I go through the days. For lunches, I use green salad as the base and pile vegetables, eggs, nuts and left-overs on top.

If you are cooking for a family your task is certainly more complicated, but your children can benefit from learning positive habits. It's hard to believe that one day, soon, they will be in their forties and maybe struggling with their weight. You will do them a great service if they see how a kitchen is managed for healthy habits.

The joy of eating at home, aside from the pleasures of cooking, is that you have control and know exactly what's going into your mouth. And, it's comforting to know that my kitchen can always offer wholesome, nutritious food if I have a few bags of whole grains and beans in the pantry. I don't hit that food emergency of having nothing in the house.

HABIT #8
SNACK OFTEN

**Keep your body running comfortably
all day long with healthy snacks
Plan ahead to avoid junk food
and say "No" to empty calories
Don't skip meals**

One of the best tricks to maintain your weight loss is to learn to make healthy choices about snacks and then to snack often.

Snacking is not having a meal. It's a micro-meal. A snack is a portion controlled, calorie-aware, small amount to eat that will make you feel comfortable for two to three hours. The intention is not to be filled up. The intention is to add a limited amount of fuel to your system so you tame your cravings, can focus on your work and feel energized. If you learn to snack smartly, you will feel comfortable all day, every day.

I snack all the time, throughout the day. It stabilizes my blood sugar, keeps my metabolism charged up and keeps me from feeling deprived. And snacking keeps me from feeling so hungry that I do something stupid.

The key is to know what you're doing and plan ahead. You should have a mental list of which foods make safe, smart snacks and then take steps to provide them for yourself. It's also important that you remove bad choices from your food environment.

Let's take a closer look.

WHY SNACKING IS GOOD FOR YOU

Skipping meals is NEVER a good idea. If you keep your blood sugar humming at a constant level, without strong dips from not eating, or strong spikes from choosing a sugar snack, you will feel good, satisfied and confident about your ability to make wise food choices during the day.

It's best to eat every three hours. Foods with fiber and protein will sustain you the longest. Avoid simple carbohydrates like sweetened foods because they metabolize so fast and will leave you jumpy and hungry within a short amount of time.

Keeping your blood sugar stable also helps control mood swings, and goodness knows we have enough of those. Don't sabotage yourself into feeling stressed, anxious and uncomfortable when your blood sugar swings down. Be prepared to snack and keep yourself satisfied.

I will most often eat raw vegetables, fruit, or whole grain crackers. The best snacks include a protein and a complex carbohydrate.

Here are recommended snacks:

Be very careful about portion control. This is a MICRO-MEAL, a bridge between larger meals.

- Slices of apple or orange
- ½ Cup of Greek yogurt. Plain. Add a teaspoon of honey, maple syrup, or sugar but don't go overboard.
- Almonds and whole grain crackers
- 1 oz of cheese and ½ cup raw vegetables
- Peanut butter and whole grain crackers
- Peanut butter and half a banana
- Unsalted pistachio meats and half an apple
- Unsweetened yogurt with granola (watch the hidden sugar)
- Fresh vegetables dipped in hummus or Greek tzatziki dip
- Chicken wrapped in lettuce. Eat as much lettuce as you like.
- One hard-boiled egg

- ½ Cup of cottage cheese

- A cup of clear soup and a slice of whole grain bread. (No butter.)

What you don't see here are sweetened coffee drinks! Stay away from the elaborate, whipped cream topped fantasy drinks at Starbucks. Yes, they're tempting but they are LOADED with sugar. If you drink coffee during the day, as I do, learn to not sweeten it. This will take a while but your taste will change.

Some people need to schedule snacks by the clock. That's fine. Try to not let more than 3 hours go by without having something nutritious to eat.

We all love to crunch, chew and suck

If you're like me, your mouth wants to move. I'll do almost anything to keep my mouth moving. I chew sugarless gum (and keep a supply in my purse and car), and sip constantly on some kind of fluid. It seems as though my mouth is always doing something.

Don't pretend that your mouth can be still if you're used to nibbling all the time. Making your mouth crunch or swallow is like an itch that needs to be scratched. Just plan ahead and make adjustments so you make healthy choices. You can keep your mouth active all day with just a little preparation. That way, you can satisfy your oral needs and still control your weight. Yes, you can do it!

Remember that some tastes are acquired. You may not like raw carrots, celery or bell peppers at the start of the effort to shift your tastes, but if you are diligent and eat a few raw vegetables every day for a snack, after about a month you will start to accept and look forward to them as part of your daily routine.

For more information about how you can reset your taste preferences, even if you think it will never happen, see *Part One: Start by Learning Why You are Unique*. It explains how taste preferences are established in childhood and what you need to do as an adult to adjust to new tastes.

Falling in love with whole grain crackers

Thank you, whole grain crackers! I really credit whole grain crackers as one of the primary tools that helped me change my eating habits for healthy weight control. I stopped eating pretzels and chips of any kind. Bye, bye, Cheetos!

I do eat whole grain crackers frequently but I rarely eat bread. A cracker is built-in portion control that really helps me control my carbohydrate intake. Five or six crackers is enough for a satisfying quick snack when I'm really in a rush.

Be sure to read the nutrition labels! Many crackers for sale nationally are really empty calories, made from refined flours and filled with sweeteners and oils. Avoid these just as rigorously as you would avoid donuts.

Crackers have crunch, which I never get tired of. The mouth action is an important part of the pleasure of eating, and whole grain crackers deliver. There are always two or three boxes in my kitchen or at my desk, and I shop for extras to keep in my pantry. I do love salt (and, fortunately, have the low blood pressure to tolerate salty snacks) but if you need to be careful about salt, be alert.

If you are shopping at the large super market chains, it may be hard to find a good selection of whole grain crackers aside from the Wasa brand, which most of the big stores carry. Consider making a trip to Costco, Whole Foods or a health food store once a month to stock up. Rice cakes made from organic brown rice are a good alternative. The Lundberg brand is popular where I live and their rice cakes are always in my cupboard.

A box of whole grain crackers is a good investment. You will get three to five days of snacks for less than $5.00.

Here are my favorite cracker brands:

- Blue Diamond Almonds Nut-Thins (Available at most supermarkets)

- Wasa whole grain (Available at most supermarkets)

- Akmak (Available at most supermarkets)

- Mary's Gone Crackers (You can get these at Costco)

- Doctor's in the Kitchen (You can get these at Whole Foods)

Drinking hot fluids helps, too

Keep something to drink at your side whenever possible. Carry a water bottle if you're moving around. If you are mostly in one place, a cup of something warm really helps.

I always have a cup of unsweetened coffee, tea or hot water with lemon at my side whenever I'm at my desk. The good news it that refilling the cup gets me up to stretch my legs! Being in the habit of sipping an unsweetened warm beverage has helped, helped, helped me control my cravings to eat more and has given me a substitute mouth satisfaction. Yes, that's three "helped". It's a good habit to learn.

Thank you, sugarless gum

Chewing gum was considered to be a rude, crude habit when I was a child. I still feel mildly uncomfortable about chewing gum in public. I would never chew gum in a professional business setting or meeting. But, putting a piece of gum in my mouth is the first thing I do in a car, sometimes before I put on my seat belt! I make sure that I always have a pack of gum in my purse and in the car and I keep a supply in my kitchen cabinet. Sugarless gum is a basic for me!

Personally, I prefer the sharp mint flavors and find that a piece of gum also satisfies my urge to eat sweets. Buying the gum that comes in a hard shell is a particularly good substitute for candies.

Do you run into convenience stores loaded with tempting bags of chips and sweets? Do you walk past displays of packaged snacks? Already having something in your mouth is a helpful tool to resist them. I don't know the neuroscience or if any studies have been done about this, but speaking from my personal experience, if my mouth is already active and moving, foods that I see casually walking by are so much less tempting.

If impulsively buying snack foods is a contributing factor to your weight gain, try chewing sugarless gum!

Healthy snacking is all about planning ahead

It's critical to plan ahead. Buy healthy snacks so you are ready when you're hungry. You can make better decisions about what goes into your mouth if you think about it ahead of time. Don't rely on being spontaneous and having self-control on instant demand.

Many snacks that are healthy for you will keep without spoiling for a while. Nuts, for example. Whole grain crackers. Vegetables like carrots, bell peppers, sugar snap peas. Apples will last in a bowl on your counter for two weeks.

No one in their right mind would advise you to snack on empty calories, fast food, sweets or other junk. That said, these can be hard to avoid, especially if you're at work. At home, you can avoid them by simply NOT BUYING junky snack foods. You can do this! Keep your hand off those packages in the store. Any store. Do not buy junk.

Any time you're tempted to reach for a junky snack, press your thumbnail into the fleshy part of a fingertip. Press hard. Turn away and don't look. You can also squeeze one of your earlobes, look away and keep squeezing. Or, you can reach down and rub your knee. Use physical touch to turn your thoughts away. You will be distracted and the desire to reach for that item will pass. And don't forget the sugarless gum.

At work, you will need to do a little more planning to be successful. Keep a supply of whole grain crackers and snack bags of almonds in your personal drawer. If food on display is allowed at your work, put a bowl of apples and oranges on your desk to visually reinforce your commitment to not eat junk. Plus, fruit is colorful and attractive. It will please your co-workers and help forge your public identity as someone who cares about fitness.

At my house, we have apples and oranges on the counter at all times. I use the apples in my morning hot whole grain cereal and I peel an orange when I feel like having something sweet. Every time I walk into the kitchen fresh fruit is a constant reminder, that I can eat snacks and still control my weight. Apples, in particular, are such a beautiful shape and color. It is a pleasure just to have them around.

Planning ahead strengthens your commitment to take good care of yourself.

You're worth it.

Don't eat chips. Really. Just don't.

Ok, chips are everywhere. Bags of salty goodness. We all love the crunch. But, you can break the chip habit. Don't buy them for any reason in any size bag. The first few weeks will be tough, but after a while, you'll stop feeling drawn to them because, frankly, they're lousy for you. There's nothing good at all in that bag except the crunch.

Do you use chips to scoop up dip? First, consider preparing vegetables like cucumber slices or bell pepper strips to dip. Then, because that dip is probably full of mayonaise or something fatty, consider not dipping and just eating the vegetables. Personally, I love guacamole, and have to be very careful with portion control. For me, the best solution is to have two scoops at most, then stand on the other side of the room.

Carry "safe" snacks in your purse along with water

Nuts are perfect for carrying in your purse. They keep, don't leak, and are very filling. My favorites are almonds. I also take fresh apple slices with me frequently.

If I know that I'm going to be busy all day and don't have a reliable place to get lunch, I take an energy bar with me, one that I have carefully read the label and know it's not full of sugars. I am not a connoisseur of energy bars but I'll eat one especially if I'm on the run. I buy the ones that are high in protein, and always have a supply ready to grab on my way out the door.

Watch out for trail mix. It can be full of unnecessary fats and often includes candy. Read the ingredients carefully and chose a trail mix with nuts, seeds and unsweetened dried fruit.

Can you nibble on cut vegetables?

You often see the advice to pre-cut vegetables and fruit like apples, carrots and celery. You will get a lot of mouth action and be able to eat as much as you'd like. Fresh vegetables are very low-density for calories: lots of volume, high-fiber, high-water content, few calories. Personally, I love cucumbers, which taste marvelous with a sprinkle of salt and dill.

For anyone who loves crunch and salt, swinging over from chips to fresh vegetables just takes some planning ahead. Cut fresh vegetables aren't available on every corner like chips are. But, vegetables are colorful, feel great in your mouth, and keep well for the day in a baggie—if you plan ahead.

12 TIPS TO MAKE SNACKING ON FRESH VEGETABLES AND FRUIT WORK FOR YOU	
Tip #1	Leave a cutting board and sharpened knife out on your counter, ready to go. I keep one out at all times so it's easy to reach for an apple and slice it up.
Tip #2	Consider putting the vegetables at eye level in your refrigerator instead of in the lower vegetable drawers. That way, they'll be the first thing you see when you look inside.
Tip #3	Buy the little carrots, ready to eat.
Tip #4	Look for stores in your neighborhood with a good produce section with a variety of pre-cut vegetables. Buy these for snacks instead of chips. You can open the bag and add salt if you're OK to eat salty foods.
Tip #5	Spend $10 for re-sealable plastic containers to store vegetables you peel and chop so they're ready to go.
Tip #6	Bite into a whole red or green bell pepper just like an apple. It requires no cutlery and is surprisingly filling.
Tip #7	Try long English cucumbers which don't need to be peeled, but don't wait more than three days to eat them. They don't keep well, unlike carrots which will last for weeks in the fridge. If you can find the mini cucumbers, these are wonderful snacks.
Tip #8	Use Romaine lettuce leaves as a wrap for leftovers. It's like a lettuce burrito.
Tip #9	Sugar snap peas are becoming more widely available. They are wonderfully crunchy and you eat the whole pod.
Tip #10	Tangerines easy to peel, fun to eat with children and delicious. Look for "Cuties" in the fruit section.
Tip #11	Steam broccoli florets in the microwave, dust them with salt or your favorite spice mix and have a bag waiting in the fridge. You can snack on these alone, or use them to top a salad.
Tip #12	Combine fresh vegetables with a healthy dipping sauce for a snack if you're watching TV. They're prettier than a bowl of popcorn!

Could you just snack and avoid a full meal?

Well, it's true: I do it all the time. I always have a good breakfast to start the day, but sometimes I have multiple snacks during the day and don't have a defined lunch. If I'm alone, working late at night, I'll have small snacks over the course of the evening and skip a full-sized dinner.

I am in no way advocating this as a lifestyle. Sharing a meal with your family or friends is preferable in every possible way to snacking alone. I'm just saying that eating multiple, small healthy snacks instead of a larger meal has worked for me without damaging my efforts to control my weight.

Just keep a tally on your calorie counts. If you have four healthy snacks for 150 calories each, it's still 600 calories. And, as always, pay attention to where those calories come from. Calories from simple carbohydrates (junk food, candy) will work against you, as explained in other chapters. Snack calories should never come from sugars or simple carbohydrates!

SNACKS AND THE FOOD ENVIRONMENT. EATING HERE, THERE, EVERYWHERE!

When I was a child in New York City in the 1950's, we were taught that it was bad manners to eat in public except at a restaurant. You just didn't see people eating walking down the street, in their cars or at their desks. The rules for good behavior in public were so much stronger then. Women wore skirts and heels at work, not pants. My father always wore a hat as part of his suit. Our family ate dinner together every night, without fail. On Sunday nights, we went to my grandmother's house and she made dinner there.

Going out to a restaurant was a special occasion! MacDonald's and the concept of fast food didn't exist yet. Outside of cereals, crackers, candy bars, and soup cans, there was very little packaged food compared to today.

These days, Americans eat everywhere, in part because packaged food for snacks seem to be available everywhere. Ninety-six percent of pharmacies sell snack food! Gift shops, dress shops, gas stations, book stores, health clubs—it seems that snacks are for sale nearly anywhere there's a cash register.

When food is visually abundant, our appetites are continually stimulated. We want what we see in front of us.

And then there are the ads, constantly pushing fast food chains and sweetened sodas. Just for the fun of it, try counting the ads you see tomorrow, in an ordinary day, on billboards, on television, in magazines. You'll be amazed how many you can count!

From home-cooked meals to fast food chains in my lifetime: A little American history

The closest thing to fast food when I was a child was the automat. Horn and Hardart was an automat chain in New York City that exemplified everything modern about the 1950's. Chrome was everywhere. All surfaces gleamed in the bright, fluorescent light. Plates of food were displayed behind glass and chrome cabinets with individual doors for each plate. You put in a nickel and could lift the door for a piece of apple pie. I loved going there as a child

In the 1950's, Horn and Hardart was serving 500,000 people every day. For about $1.00, you could get a pretty decent meal. And…you could chose exactly the plate you wanted. When we visited my father's office in Manhattan, I always wanted to eat at the automat. The sparkle of the shiny metal surfaces and the freedom—I could make my own choice! It was intoxicating for a child.

And, the automat was a novelty and introduced a brand-new concept of fast food. Before the automat, eating out meant ordering your food and then you waited to be served, whether you were at a café or an elegant restaurant. But at the automat, everything was precooked so the food was in your hands as soon as you made your decision.

Automats only lasted for about twenty years before they were swept away by the popularity of fast food outlets.

Home cooking is no longer the rule. How did eating food cooked outside the home become so popular?

Eating in restaurants used to be a special treat for most families because meals not prepared at home were generally very expensive. It was a special occasion when my parents took their three children out to eat. I know families who never went to restaurants in the 1950's and 1960's because dining out cost too much money for their family budgets.

In the 1970's, two things happened that made eating out more popular for American families:

- Thanks to government support, US farm production soared in the 1970's. Suddenly, American farmers were producing more food and calories than the population could possibly eat. At the same time, mega-national food companies had to find new food products to use up all this abundance. Food supplies became cheaper.

- Fast food chains sprang up around the country starting in the 1970's, making it so much easier to buy ready-made food. The price and the convenience persuaded hardworking Americans to accept take-out meals as a normal way of life in the 1970's. Widespread advertising helped inexpensive food outlets to gain national traction. Today, driven by demand, 75% of Americans live within a three-mile radius of a McDonald's.

Today, food writers and nutrition experts urge us to cook meals at home. It's not just what we're cooking, it's that the whole concept of eating a family meal cooked at home has become a cause which needs support from leading thinkers. This alone would have been an alien thought to most of our grandparents for whom cooking at home, 365 days a year was normal.

DON'T TRUST SLOGANS ON THE PACKAGING
ESPECIALLY FOR SNACK FOODS
Read the ingredients and nutrition labels

Did you know that over 20,000 new food products are launched every year? Who buys this stuff? Could you be persuaded to buy a food product because of marketing slogans. For most people, the answer is "yes". Nobody is immune unless you learn something about sales psychology. Millions of dollars are being spent in a frantic effort to convince you to buy snacks, drinks, packaged foods.

Unless you buy your food exclusively at farmers' markets, you are spending money and supporting multi-national food corporations. The first loyalty for these companies is to their stockholders, not to you. Think that a packaging designer really cares about your blood pressure? No. That packaging designer cares about keeping his job, winning an industry award for his box design and hoping that the food product will sell well so he'll get more work.

Food is a product that must sell. You must be persuaded to spend your dollars on any particular item. The days when most families kept a garden and farm animals are long gone. (Although backyard chickens are making a comeback!). Most people who buy their ready-made food or food supplies are the consumers at the end of a very long, industrial supply chain.

This puts you in the position of needing to trust those food companies to take care of your nutritional health. I think you'd be better off if you trusted yourself.

Beware of packaging. I spent my career as a product designer, launching successful products, and I can promise you from an insider's perspective that every possible effort is made by marketing companies to understand your shopping psychology and then manipulate you to buy their products. The color, shape, size and placement of the package all matter. The words used to attract you are chosen carefully: "Healthy" "Natural" "Whole" "Good for your heart". Forget all of this. JUST READ THE INGREDIENT AND NUTRITION LABELS. If you don't understand what's in the product or see sugar and high fructose corn syrup high on the list of ingredients, don't even think about buying it. Put it back on the shelf.

Trust yourself. Don't trust the marketing people.

The point is worth repeating. If you eat fast food, pre-cooked food or packaged food for most of your daily diet, you are transferring the ability to control the ingredients to someone else. This means that you owe it to yourself to be hyper-vigilant about what is in the food you are eating.

Why trust someone who doesn't really care about you, the customer, and cares more about making money? You really can't. You must take responsibility for learning what's in the food you buy if you want to control your weight. You must be observant, ask questions and probably do some research on the internet.

Just because a product claims to be healthy doesn't mean it's a healthy choice for you. Flavored Greek yogurt, for example. This wildly popular product is flooding the market with fruit-flavored cups of non-fat yogurt that can have nearly as much sugar as ice cream. Yet, if you ask the average woman if it's a healthy choice, she will have been programmed by the advertising and packaging to say "yes". How can yogurt, which has been sweetened like a dessert, be a healthy snack for people trying to lose or control their weight? Read the ingredients, then trust yourself to decide what's healthy for you.

HABIT #9
ENJOY AT LEAST ONE NON-CALORIC PLEASURE EVERY DAY

Stimulate all your senses:
Touch, smell, sight, hearing, not just taste
Enjoy your body: Have more orgasms!

Our bodies have astonishing sensual abilities. We hear beautiful music, smell subtle aromas, touch soft fabrics, see sunsets, taste interesting flavors and have orgasms. In my heavyweight years, I often forgot about using all of my five senses and, instead, really focused on what was happening in my mouth. I enjoyed the tastes and textures of food and how full my stomach felt after a big meal. I was going through life like a giant, hungry mouth.

One of the best things I ever did for myself was to enrich my life by paying daily attention to giving pleasure to each of my senses. It wasn't expensive. In fact, pleasuring your senses can be entirely free—you can smell the flowers at the supermarket without buying them, or run your fingers softly across the warm skin of your shoulder. I would make a daily inventory, touch-smell-sight-hearing-taste, and make sure that each sense had at least one special moment.

I encourage you to engage all of your senses as part of your weight control program. Knowing that you can have pleasure, great pleasure, reliable pleasure from something besides eating seems obvious, but unless you actively commit to seeking out pleasure for your senses, it can get lost in your daily rush. We are certainly going to talk about orgasms—and I hope that got your attention—but all of your senses deserve your focus.

Committing to sensual pleasure will reinforce your positive feelings about your body

Eating alone in a room used to be a great source of pleasure for me. I particularly love ice cream and would savor mouthfuls, especially mocha chip, my favorite flavor. I'd roll the chips around on my tongue, feeling the sweet creamy fluid slip down my throat. Yes, it was sensual.

I relied on the sense of taste for most of my pleasure, and ignored the rich experiences available from my other senses. I should have paid more attention to touch, sight, hearing and smell which not only would have made my days so much more enjoyable, but it would have helped to put some perspective on the undue emphasis I had been placing on what was happening in my mouth.

Hopefully, you are lucky and your hearing, eyesight, sense of smell and nerve endings in your fingers are all working as they should. If how much pleasure you are receiving is dominated by taste and you are over-looking your other senses, it's time now to start reinforcing your ability to have constant pleasures with your body.

It takes practice to break away from being dominated by mouth focus. You've had years of being able to trust this source of pleasure and comfort. It will take some time and practice to build up that level of trust for your other senses, but it can be done. And, what fun and enjoyment awaits you in the process!

This is truly a win-win, only good-results-are-possible process. By adding sensual pleasures to your menu of weight control techniques, you can only enrich your life experience and contribute to your sense of happiness.

Deep breathing clears the mind, sets the stage

We'll go through each sense, but let's get started with one of my favorite sensual tricks that only takes a moment, and is absolutely free: deep breathing. You can do this in any position at any time of day. I always do a deep breathing session, as I'm laying quietly in bed, getting ready to go to sleep.

Here's how to do deep breathing:

Close your eyes. Place your fingertips lightly on your ribcage, under your breasts. Listen for 10 seconds to the sounds around you. Swallow. Slowly, take in the deepest breath you can, imagining the air going down to the bottom of your lungs. Feel your ribcage expand. Hold your breath for 5 seconds and be surprised at how your ribs expand further. Exhale slowly through your mouth, listening to the air escape your body. Swallow. Take 3 regular breaths.

Repeat for a total of 3 deep breaths.

TOUCH: THE QUEEN OF SENSES

Your hands are the best and easiest opportunity to transfer attention away from your mouth. From washing and feeling the warm water run through your fingers, to stroking your thighs through the texture of your clothes, you can always distract yourself with a pleasurable sensation.

- Lay your fingers on your cheek. Notice the difference in temperature. Run your thumb softly across your jaw then trace the outline of your lips. Let your index finger start at your inner eyebrow, following your brow then explore the outline and folds of your ear. Scratch behind your ear and feel the sharpness of your nail against your soft skin.

- Do you like your bedsheets? If you can afford it, buy new sheets with a higher thread count. Climb into bed with bare legs. Swing your legs gently back and forth, feeling the top sheet slide against your knees. Think about the wonderful things that can happen between sheets. Reach up to your pillowcase. Rub its edge between your fingers.

- For your shower or bath, use a new sponge or cloth. Feel the warm water cascade across your back. Lift your arms and shake in the water's flow, feeling how the spray changes with your movement.

- Treat yourself to a massage.

- Try not to think about your shoes if they hurt your feet! We want pleasurable touch, not pain!

- Walk barefoot across your home or garden. Close your eyes and curl your toes.

- Take a walk and feel the breeze on your skin.

- Choose a silky or soft neck scarf. Don't miss the opportunity to notice how it feels on your throat.

In fact, touch is a big part of eating. We love to touch food with our fingers, grasp it, move it to our mouth, feel it on our lips. Feeling your warm, wet tongue on your lips is a non-caloric pleasure. Run your tongue behind your upper lip, keeping your tongue soft. Then, repeat with your tongue stiff and hard. Enjoy feeling the difference.

Here are some other suggestions:

- Consider getting a cat or dog. Nothing will add more vibrancy to your daily life than touching a warm and furry pet who enthusiastically wants your touch. If you can't have a pet, consider getting a furry pillow to stroke.

- Garden and appreciate handling the plants and soil. Feel the sunlight and breeze on your arms.

- Take ceramic lessons and play with clay.

- Knit or crochet and enjoy the yarns and the smooth feel of the needles.

- Sit in a hot tub with spa jets.

- Go clothes shopping and revel in the textures of fabrics.

- Buy a new hairbrush.

- Have a manicure-pedicure.

HEARING: THE GATEWAY TO MUSIC AND LANGUAGE

Hearing is the easiest sense for me to take for granted and I have to force myself to stop and listen. I envy musicians who live surrounded by beautiful and exciting sounds.

Try these tips to increase your awareness of what you hear:

- When you first wake up, dedicate 20 seconds to listening to your breathing. Then press your ear into the pillow and listen for your heartbeat.

- Sing.

- If you're a mother, close your eyes and just listen to your children breathe while they're sleeping.

- Pick a radio station you wouldn't ordinarily listen to and try some new music for five minutes.

- If you are familiar with classical music, chose your favorite symphony and buy a recording. I recommend Brahms First Symphony, my personal favorite. Listen with your eyes closed. Better yet, go to a concert of live music.

- Stand still outside and listen. Try to get to a park once a week to listen to bird song.

- Tap your foot and create a rhythm.

- Put a bell or chime on your key ring.

- Go to a busy store and try to identify any accents or foreign languages.

- Stand in a doorway with people walking by and close your eyes. Try to identify the gender and age of the people walking by.

Interesting sounds and rhythms are all around us. If you're fortunate to be musical, perhaps you don't need additional advice on how to enhance your appreciation for what you hear! For the rest of us, stopping to spend a few minutes every day to focus on our hearing, is a worthy use of time.

Here are some other suggestions:

- Seek out water sounds—go sit by a fountain when you eat lunch.

- Listen to your friends talk with your eyes closed.

- Whistle.

- Whisper.

- Count how many sounds you can make when your fingers touch each other. Snap, rub, clap, shake. Build up rhythms with your sounds.

SMELL: THE SWEET AND SOUR PLAYGROUND

The human nose is an incredibly sensitive instrument but it doesn't always age well. As we get older, our sense of smell diminishes. Plus, when we get used to specific aromas in a specific setting, we are no longer conscious of them. Sometimes, that's a good thing! My mother loved cats. Lots of cats. I never noticed that our home smelled like a cat box, but my friends often mentioned it when they came to visit.

Here are ideas to identify times in your day when you can add the pleasure of smell:

- After you brush your teeth at night, rub a little scented lotion or oil on the tip of your nose. Try eucalyptus oil.

- Put a scented mini-pillow in your underwear drawer. Lavender is the classic scent.

- Ask for scented powder for a birthday present then lightly dust yourself before you go to bed.

- Do you like perfume? Start a perfume shelf in your bathroom. At the cosmetic counters of better department stores, you can ask for perfume samples.

- Buy a beautifully scented soap then use it in the morning to wash your hands.

- Light a scented candle. For a really strong scent, light incense.

- Smell your farts. Yes, we all enjoy our own...it's a guilty pleasure.

- Smell under your nails. Mine smell like toe jam. Time to wash!

- Chew mint gum and notice how the smell goes up the back of your throat.

- If you're a mother, bury your face in your children's hair and take a deep breath.

- Yes, stop and smell the roses.

Sour and unpleasant odors grab our attention. We usually try to move away as quickly as possible. The unpleasant experience is still useful to remind us that our sense of smell can be powerful. I've heard that smells can trigger memories faster than visual or auditory clues. That's certainly true for me. Smells from my childhood carry me right back. Is this true for you?

Here are some more suggestions:

- In a kitchen or restaurant, close your eyes and try to identify as many aromas as possible.

- Enjoy wine tasting.

- Sample cheeses with your eyes closed.

- If your purse is leather, put your nose inside and take a deep breath.

- Rub a leaf on your palm and smell.

- Sniff the armpits of your sweaters and jackets.

- If you have a sexual partner, run your nose up and down his/her body to find the place that smells best to you.

- Open your front door, close your eyes, and try to identify 5 smells.

SIGHT: FOR MOST OF US, OUR PRIMARY GUIDE TO THE WORLD

Like many people, I am a visual learner and absolutely rely on my sight for receiving most of my information about the world. But, I don't usually think of seeing as a sensual pleasure unless the experience is coupled with emotion. Seeing a poignant photograph that tells a story can make me cry. The vibrant colors of garden flowers can make my heart leap for joy.

Here's how you can use seeing as a pleasure tool to reinforce your good weight control habits.

- Create a vision board of positive images. See yourself as fit and healthy by gathering images of healthy women doing activities you would like to share. Bicycling, climbing a tree, surfing or summiting a mountain, pictures of strong women who can be role models will help keep you focused. You can physically tear out magazine pictures or create this on Pinterest.

- Enjoy colors. Pick a color for the day, notice and comment to yourself when you see it.

- Buy new underpants. OK, this sounds goofy, but each time you go to the bathroom, you pull down your pants and will see something you enjoy. I am secretly enjoying purple underpants this year. When I go to the ladies room, I have a private smile and moment of enjoyment when I see that rich, purple color. And...it reminds me to stay on track with my weight control program.

- Paint your bedroom a color you enjoy. Take your time choosing paint samples, spreading out the swatches and playing with the different shades.

- Go clothes shopping! You don't have to buy. Pick a color, for example, blue, and count how many different shades you can find.

- Go to a garden center and look closely at the shapes of the flowers. Walk under a tree and look up at the light coming through the branches.

- Keep fresh flowers in your house if you can afford it.

- If you have an aquarium, spend some time enjoying the colors and movements of the fish. Add new, colorful fish if you can.

- Go to a bookstore and enjoy book covers. Pick your favorite.

- Sit in the dark by the light of one candle. Think about the generations of people who lived by candlelight. Make a wish then blow out the candle.

- Draw a heart on your palm with warm water then watch it evaporate.

- Go to an art museum and imagine that you have painted all the pictures there. Think about the colors on the paintbrushes and how your arm would have moved while painting.

- When you go to a movie, try to think about the lighting design. How does lighting in the film direct your focus and enhance the story told by the director?

Here are some more suggestions:

- Have a manicure in a wild color.

- Buy new throw pillows for your couch or bed.

- Find a new, colorful coffee mug you really like, and use it every morning.

- Wake up early and watch the sunrise.

- Watch at least one sunset every week.

- Love the color of your towels; if you don't, replace them. Pay attention to the color as you rub the towels up your legs, across your belly and down your arms.

- Find a key ring that makes you smile every time you use your keys.

- Look for every opportunity to surround yourself with beauty.

TASTE: GREAT PLEASURE, GREAT RISK

I am going to go lightly on this section on taste because, my guess is, that you already know full-well about the pleasures your sense of taste can deliver. Overeating is not just about how great things taste, of course, but you probably don't need any further instructions on how to get pleasure from your mouth!

Let's just cover that both your taste buds and your nose's olfactory nerves are involved. Without a sense of smell, it's hard to taste much of anything, as you probably know from having a stuffy nose.

My recommendation is to practice tasting tiny portions of new flavors. Be brave! Unsweetened coffee? Unflavored yogurt? Curry? Hot sauce? A new vegetable? Flavored salts are terrific if you are allowed to enjoy salt. Think about what you can safely put in your mouth that will be a new, adventurous taste.

Your mouth is a pleasure organ and can do many other things besides taste. Crunch, lick, slurp and suck originate in your mouth and are just plain fun. OK, maybe not in polite company, but most of us love a good crunch.

Here are just a few ideas on how to expand your sense of taste:

- Cultivate a taste for tea. The choices are nearly infinite.

- Make flavored ice cubes from tea then see if you can identify them.

- Chew a cinnamon stick. It will fill your mouth with flavor...and help with bad breath!

- Put an empty teaspoon in your mouth. Can you taste the metal?

- Taste your soap.

- Try different sugarless gums until you pick a favorite.

- Explore the tastes of your own body. Put your finger in your belly button then in your mouth.

- Try edible flowers, petal by petal.

- Take a nibble of your dog's or cat's food.

- Taste a sip of water like you would fine wine. Roll it around in your mouth. Try this with warm water and again with cold water. Do you notice a difference?

- Dip a toothpick in hot sauce then touch it to your tongue. See if you can identify the area of your tongue that responds to spicy foods. Maybe it's all over!

ORGASM: A GOOD SEXUAL EXPERIENCE SHOULD BE PART OF YOUR FITNESS PROGRAM

I saved the best for last in this chapter, except that you probably skipped the rest and came here first!

When we don't feel good about our bodies because of our size and appearance, it's easy to forget that nature gave us a built-in path to pleasure. Women don't need any equipment. Just a clean hand and privacy to remind ourselves that our bodies can feel wonderful. If you have a satisfying partner, all the better!

Any woman who is committed to fitness and healthy habits should consider having an orgasm as part of her daily routine. Not only is having regular orgasms good stimulation for your organs, circulatory system and brain, but orgasms are compelling proof that your body is a trustworthy source of goodness and happiness. If you're unhappy with yourself, it's a quick fix!

Some women feel uncomfortable and ashamed of their bodies. They are so used to cringing and feeling bad about how they look and feel. Nobody needs orgasms more than women who want to gain control of their health and develop a positive body image.

Our culture of celebrity thin women doesn't make this any easier, of course. We fall into believing that thin is sexy and extra weight is a turn-off. So, if you are carrying any extra pounds, maybe you don't whole-heartedly believe that your body is sensual, attractive and capable of feeling really, really good. Why not remind yourself that you're so lucky to be alive? Run your hands across that wonderful body of yours that carried you through the day and give yourself the physical pleasure your deserve.

See that you have an orgasm every single day of the week. Make it one of your must-do habits. Talk to a therapist or counselor if you feel blocked or unsure. I sincerely hope that you move towards being able to have this basic, human pleasure and enjoyment.

If you need lubricants, vibrators or sex toys, go to the very informative and supportive Good Vibrations website. www.goodvibrations.com And, in case you didn't know, Amazon sells a full selection, too.

It's reported that women take an average of 4 minutes to masturbate to orgasm. So don't even think that you don't have enough time in your day. 4 Minutes. Really!

Be confident that your body will give you pleasure.

Go have fun!

HABIT #10
CONTROL YOUR FOOD CRAVINGS

Manage excessive food desire
and get help when you need it
Understanding willpower

Cravings, yearnings and obsessions are an everyday part of life for many people. I used to be one of them. I healed myself from being driven by uncontrolled cravings for food by asking for help, and then following recommendations and practicing over and over until new behaviors became habits. I sought help many times over the years and kept trying different things until I was able to put together a blend of techniques that worked for me.

Here are the commitments you need to learn controlling your food cravings:

- Your first commitment is to seek help and advice.

- Your second commitment is to accept that you will need to always be learning how to help yourself.

Learning new ways to control your cravings is a lifelong attitude. Just like weight control habits are lifelong behaviors, not just temporary actions. Being open to helping yourself resist temptation and cravings is an attitude that you can embrace permanently.

If you are willing to learn something new, you can protect your weight control as your body changes. (Yes, our bodies change when we age, especially those of us who are menopausal women!) Again, when we talk about "weight control", we are in a discussion about years of everyday behaviors, not a short-term weight loss diet activity burst.

Help comes in many forms. Be open to them all. Be an active learner!

For me, some help was talk therapy and hypnosis therapy; some help came from distraction tricks I learned from friends, books, weight loss programs or magazines. Other forms of help came from focusing on how to <u>strengthen willpower</u> as a skill that can be applied to many situations, not just food cravings. If you have read this far, you've noticed that strengthening willpower is a major theme of this book.

I also paid attention to what was working for my friends and family members, many of whom were also struggling to keep extra pounds off. We're a diverse group, with lots of different eating preferences and body types. I questioned them, and listened carefully if someone was having success with weight control.

In this chapter, I'm going to share what I've learned over the years and what could be applied practically to my everyday life. These techniques have worked for my friends, my family members and me. They can work for you!

But first, we need to separate food cravings into three distinct groupings:

- **Temporary temptation:** A craving that is the result of seeing something you want. You weren't thinking about that chocolate until, suddenly, you see it! Persuasive advertising teaches us to want, want, want. Sometimes, we can't control ourselves. We just want more pizza or that dessert because temptation is everywhere. Be kind to yourself, especially if you have a sweet tooth. You can learn to control your cravings!

- **Physical need:** A craving that is the result of an addiction or a metabolic condition. Examples would include alcohol and sugar.

- **Obsessive need:** A craving that is the result of a neurological or psychological condition, possibly obsessive-compulsive behavior.

In this chapter, we will focus on temporary temptation, the kind of craving you experience when you see food and start thinking about it. You will find these pages chock full of tips and tricks to help keep you from falling into temptation.

While we shouldn't ignore the pull of food addictions and serious, neurological and psychological eating disorders such as bulimia, these are topics too complex for the scope of this book. If you think that you are dealing with any of these serious conditions, please do not hesitate to get professional help.

The following discussion is based on my personal experience and observations, and is not intended to be a substitute for qualified, professional help.

DISTRACT YOUR BRAIN FROM A TEMPORARY CRAVING: TRY THESE TIPS—THEY WORK ANYTIME, ANYWHERE.

Most cravings are passing thoughts your brain presents to you as response to an environmental stimulus. For example, you have walked into the coffee lounge at your office and there's a box of donuts on the counter. Twenty seconds ago, you weren't thinking about donuts but now lustful thoughts about their deliciousness fill your head. You want one. You don't want to walk away without one.

Maybe you're at a party and there's a plate of chocolate chip cookies. Oh, how you love chocolate chip cookies. Me, too! You take one and walk across the room. But, as soon as you've swallowed the last bite, your eyes turn back to the plate. Another. Another! "Come get me," the cookies are calling.

What you need is a quick distraction

Your brain's pleasure centers are lit up and you feel driven, compulsively focused on the food you want. *The key right now is to light up another center in your brain.*

Distract yourself for one minute—just 60 seconds—and the craving will pass. And… don't forget to move away and take the temptation out of sight!

Try these 6 tricks to distract yourself:

- **TIP #1: Push your thumbnail into the soft tip of your middle finger as hard as you can.**

It hurts! Lessen your grip a little but keep pulsing your thumbnail into your soft flesh. Look at your hand. I guarantee you that if you do this for 30 seconds you will forget about that jelly donut. The nerve stimulation will override your imaginary desire.

You can also squeeze your earlobe. Hard. Turn away—don't look!— and keep squeezing. You'll be amazed at how fast you can distract yourself and recover from temptation.

- **TIP #2: Stroke anything tactile that will grab your attention.**

You always have something to touch: your lapel, the lining of your jacket pocket, jiggling your keys, fingering the sharp end of your earring—anything that will grab your attention. If I'm wearing a jacket with a zipper, I stroke my thumb over the zipper.

A friend of mine, Erica, carries a piece of soft velvet in her pocket. If she's tempted by sweet food, she'll fondle the velvet and look away until the craving passes.

Sometimes, I rub my fingers into the hair at the back of my neck and think about whether I need to brush my hair. This is a very effective way to stop thinking about food, especially if you think about your hair a lot. (Coloring, styling…it can be a big topic and useful for distraction!)

You can do any of these tactile distraction techniques and no one will notice. What you want to do is draw your attention away from the desired food, not draw attention to yourself!

- **TIP #3: Put another image in your mind, something really racy.**

The part of your brain that holds a visual image in your imagination can hold only one image at a time. Are you thinking about that chocolate bar? Well, replace it with an image of your neighbor running naked across his lawn. Shocking? I hope so.

Thinking about naked people really helps me calm cravings, especially for sweets. Do I always think about naked neighbors? No. Sometimes

I think about naked celebrities. If the craving is especially bad, I think about naked politicians and usually lose my appetite instantly!

- **TIP #4: Remind yourself about your goals. Write a few notes on a small card and keep it in your pocket.**

When you feel temptation, reach in and rub the card, thinking about how much you want to achieve your goals. If that doesn't work fast enough, take out the card and read your goals, affirming each one to yourself.

Soon, you will have programed your brain to have a positive, goal-affirming response as soon as you touch the card.

I keep a card like this in my pocket every day of the week. My goals vary over time, but reminding myself to stay positive and on track has become part of my daily life. Keeping my goals front and center and a reminder card readily available has really helped me avoid unnecessary temptation.

- **TIP #5: Focus on your teeth and tongue: Cleanse your mouth with water, gum or brushing.**

Since temptation is going to lead you to put something in your mouth, go straight to your mouth with your mind. If you're in public, run your tongue around every tooth. Take a breath for every tooth—this will really slow you down! If you can, grab a glass of water and sip it slowly. If you're at home, leave the room and go brush your teeth.

I find that chewing sugarless gum is very helpful. There's something about already having something in my mouth that makes me resist putting anything else in. Gum chewing isn't always possible, but I always carry gum in my purse and my car. I make a point of chewing gum when I go grocery shopping and find that this really helps me resist the temptation to reach for sugary foods.

Are you thinking that this is too simple? That easy techniques to help you resist food temptations can't really work? Yes, they can! But, easy techniques work better if they're part of an overall program to help you stay on track to build your willpower.

PLAN AHEAD TO AVOID TEMPTATION.
JUST DON'T GO THERE.

What you look at matters. Plan ahead to clear your field of vision from temptations.

If you plan ahead and clean up your food environment, it will be easier to avoid temptation. Set yourself up for success by removing unhealthy snack foods from your home and office as much as you can. Be willing to throw out that bag of chips! The work environment is particularly hard because you probably don't have 100% control. Ask co-workers to support you, if you can.

I am not an advocate for throwing away food. It's wasteful. But, if you have packages of processed food in your home, especially those full of sugar, fat and salt, just know that keeping these around will make it harder to build your will to resist. Every time you see them, you will have to make an active decision to eat or not. It's much better to not set yourself up to make this choice. Replace the processed, packaged snack foods in your kitchen with healthy, whole foods. See *Habit #8: Snack Often* for more tips on which snack foods to keep around you.

Avoid going places that will bring on cravings. For example, I love cookies. If I go into a good bakery, I'm in trouble, so I don't go in unless I have a mission to buy a birthday cake.

Look away! If you let your eyes linger on that box of chocolate, every minute that goes by makes it harder to resist. Pinch yourself and walk away.

KEEPING YOUR BLOOD SUGAR STEADY
HELPS YOU RESIST TEMPTATION

When your blood sugar is low, studies have shown that you are more prone to impulsive eating behavior.

Here's why: The brain needs glucose—that's its *only* energy source. (Blood sugar level is actually a measurement of the amount of glucose in your blood. For more information, see *Habit #6: Avoid Added Sugars and Sweetened Drinks*.) So, to protect itself while your blood glucose levels are falling, the brain will hold back signals from its centers that generate self-control.

Grabbing for any available food is a simple consequence of your brain registering that its energy levels are dropping. And, in our culture of readily available fast food and packaged food, full of sugar and salt, it's so easy to eat "food" that offers you nothing but empty calories and weight gain.

We've all experienced this. It's just harder to hold back from eating snack food if you're really hungry. Your impulse is to buy and eat it. Right away!

Psychologists working with people with impulse control issues look at what they're eating. High-sugar, empty calorie foods are very suspect. These cause a sharp rise in blood sugar, which is followed by a steep drop, as your pancreas, releases extra insulin to bring your glucose levels back to a healthy balance. You've heard this called an "insulin spike".

You don't have to be a diabetic to experience the effects of your blood sugar going up and down. If you struggle with impulsive eating, please do some research and do everything you can to keep your blood sugar steady.

And….be sure to talk to your doctor for more information if you're concerned about keeping your blood sugar stabilized.

UNDERSTANDING YOUR WILLPOWER: WHY IS IT HARDER TO RESIST TEMPTATION AS YOUR DAY GOES ON?

Is willpower a limited resource during the day? Yes! Let's take a look at why, and how you can preserve your willpower resources so you can resist temptation when you really need to.

It's all inside your brain, and as researchers are learning more and more each year, your brain is very sensitive to what you eat and drink, how you sleep, whether or not you exercise, and what you see and hear. And, it turns out that your willpower reserve is also sensitive to how many decisions you make during the day. Your brain can simply get tired of making decisions and choices. You can lose your ability to say "no", especially if you're physically right next to a source of temptation.

Willpower, or as it's sometimes called "self-control", is the product of interactions inside the prefrontal cortex of your brain—the front brain section responsible for making decisions. It's not just one spot, but a complex relationship between three different areas, discovered by scientists mapping brain regions.

These three areas are incredibly powerful forces in our daily lives—they store and control our goals and desires. These parts of the brain make you feel responsible and keep you on task.

But, do these three areas operate at peak efficiency all day long? Sadly, no. They get tired and "run out of gas". Of course this isn't a scientific way of explaining the process! For more information, see *PART FIVE: Resources for Learning More* for recommended books by scientists and science reporters on the subject of willpower.

Basically, researchers are finding that your willpower is like a muscle that gets tired from making decisions. You are presented with food choices, and the sweet, fatty or salty flavors call to you. You make good choices for breakfast, do fairly well for lunch, but by late afternoon, you're having a harder time. And then, you wreck your whole day of good eating habits at dinner or by continuing to eat crazy stuff into the night. Bedtime comes and you resolve to do better tomorrow, but the pattern repeats itself. That's what happened to me.

In my life, this explains why I would often binge-eat at night, especially after 9:00 pm. I already had dinner, but I just couldn't resist eating pretzels until the bag was empty, or ice cream until I hit the bottom of the carton. I didn't have trouble keeping my resolutions to not overeat when the day started, but all my resistance had faded away by nighttime.

Understanding decision fatigue: It's real.

We live in a culture of continued stimulation and we need to make hundreds of decisions every day. What do I wear today? What am I eating for breakfast? Do we put regular or premium gas in the car? Which lane or line is faster? Shopping. School. Work. Money. Planning. Social media. Advertisements. Television commercials. Choices. Choices. Choices….

Roy F. Baumeister is a leading research psychologist who studies self-control and coined the term "decision fatigue". With the science journalist, John Tierney, he wrote an excellent book, *Willpower: Rediscovering the Greatest Human Strength*. It would be well worth your time to buy a copy and read it.

Here are two critical findings from scientific research on willpower:

Finding #1: Each individual has a finite amount of willpower, which gets used up through your actions and decisions during the day.

Finding #2: All willpower comes from the same place. You cannot store willpower for eating or willpower for exercising or working hard in separate allotments. You have only one mental storage of willpower and you draw from it for everything you do.

When Baumeister and his colleagues studied people in multiple different scenarios and circumstances, they found the same result: when more decisions were required over time to resist temptation, people became less decisive and weaker at resisting temptations. Their reserves of will power became worn out.

So, what does this mean for you? It means that the more decisions you make, the more depleted your willpower reserves become, until you can sleep and rest your brain so it can replenish itself.

There are many practical applications in your life. Notice, for example, how you react if you walk slowly through a supermarket, really studying the choices on the shelves. Do you do more impulse shopping at the end of your trip or at the beginning? At the end, for most of us. There's a reason why the cashier's counters are filled with candies. How often do you reach for a treat that you would have resisted just fifteen minutes ago?

Your brain is very sensitive to environmental stimulus. Visual, auditory, smell, touch. Our brains are marvelously responsive. Advertisers count on our sense of sight to stimulate desire. See food—want it. If we're practicing weight control, we simply can't eat everything we see. We are forced to resist/reject so much of the food that comes before us. This leads quickly to decision fatigue and lack of resistance.

BUT....there is hope! Believe it or not YOU CAN TRAIN your brain to ignore temptation. It takes practice but you can learn the habit of controlling your cravings.

And it starts with a good night's sleep.

After a good sleep, your brain is rested and your willpower is at its peak.

Your body simply needs sleep for all systems to work properly, and the brain system controlling willpower is no exception. When you wake up after a full night's sleep, your neocortex can operate at its optimal level. You start the day with a "full tank" of willpower.

With each and every decision you make, you draw down on that tank. If you are surrounded by food choices you need to make in the morning and then again at lunchtime, your "willpower tank" has started running down. For snack time in the afternoon, if you have to resist cookies or sugar soda, you spend more from your tank. Until finally, you reach the end of your day at home, and there's ice cream in the freezer that you absolutely can't resist any more.

That was my story. I would exhaust my willpower during the day, working, helping my kids, running our household, and at night, even after a full dinner, food temptations would call to me and I couldn't resist. The ice cream in our freezer would call to me. I would start with a spoonful, put the container back, walk around the room, telling myself that a spoonful was enough. But, I'd be back. And then, after a few spoonfuls more, I would surrender to the carton and consume the ice cream until I hit the cardboard on the bottom. Truly, I had a food obsession. And that's why I went for help—which worked! We'll talk more about this more in a few pages.

CONTROL YOUR CRAVINGS BY STRENGTHENING YOUR WILLPOWER

The good news is that it's possible to learn to protect your willpower reserves so you have self-control when you need it for food cravings.

It starts by making a commitment to learning what you need to do. It also starts by believing that what you are doing is positive: you're protecting and strengthening your willpower. Instead of thinking that resisting a craving is a negative action (saying "no"), you can learn to reposition your choice as a positive: "I'm strengthening my willpower". Making this attitude change helps create positive habits. The more you are positive, the more encouragement and success you'll experience.

This is so important, it should be repeated:

Shift your attitude away from the negative "I can't have that" to the positive "I am making my willpower stronger".

The more times you convert a negative experience into a positive one, the easier it will be to resist temptation. Soon, instead of feeling pulled by temptation, you will find it easy to ignore it while feeling good about yourself because you have reinforced a positive attitude. You will feel positive instead of deprived.

Being positive really works!

And…sooner than you think, you will spend less energy ignoring temptation because when you make the same decision over and over again, it eventually becomes automatic and requires very little effort on your part. Which means very little willpower is used up, and you protect your reserves for more demanding tasks.

So, although resisting a flood of food temptations can seem overwhelming at first, if you break it down to mastering one temptation at a time, you will experience success and be encouraged.

You can manage this! Let's take a closer look.

12 TIPS TO PROTECT & STRENGTHEN YOUR WILLPOWER RESERVES	
Tip #1	When you are first starting to protect your willpower supply, be very vigilant about decision fatigue. Try to minimize the decisions you need to make at the start of your day. Do as much planning ahead as possible the night before. Chose your clothes and lay them out, ready for the morning. Make and pack your lunch so it's waiting for you. Decide what you're going to have for breakfast before you go to bed.
Tip #2	Get the best sleep you possibly can. Remember, the neocortex in your brain simply needs to rest! Seven hours is best for most people. You will have more willpower first thing in the morning after a good night's sleep than at any other time of the day.
Tip #3	After you wake up, try to establish and follow a morning routine. You can minimize the number of decisions you make first thing in the morning, if you know what's expected. If you have children to get ready, this is especially important.
Tip #4	Keep your blood sugar steady during the day. Start with a breakfast of protein and high fiber to sustain your blood sugar at stable levels throughout the morning. Never, never NEVER start the day with sugary foods to avoid a sugar crash, which will lead you to grab whatever food you see in front of you.
Tip #5	Don't skip lunch. If you must eat at your desk, plan ahead to have high-fiber foods.
Tip #6	Avoid people who have lousy eating habits if you possibly can. If these are co-workers, don't follow them to the vending machines. If it's your family members who want to binge on pizza and beer, gather up your courage and learn to talk to them about supporting you in learning new habits so you can control your weight.
Tip #7	Don't drink too much alcohol—this will impair your judgment. And, wine, beer and cocktails are full of sugar and calories.
Tip #8	Do your best to simplify and streamline how many decisions you need to make during the day. Being overloaded is not to be taken lightly. It can exhaust your willpower supply quickly and even put your health at risk from stress. Do everything you can to research and implement ways to simplify the decisions you're facing. (A few quick suggestions: List making, time management tools, delegation, asking for help, meditation, and regular exercise.)
Tip #9	Set smaller goals and practice them. Example: "I will not buy ice cream this week" instead of "I'll never eat dessert again!" Large goals are overwhelming. Small goals are manageable.

Tip #10	Create a positive affirmation to say when you are faced with food temptation. Example: "I'm building my willpower", instead of "I can't have that chocolate cake". Try as much as possible to avoid negative statements and find a positive way to describe your decision.
Tip #11	Practice, practice, practice. New habits take many, many repetitions to take root, but each time you practice a new behavior, it gets a little easier. It may not be obvious at first, but keep practicing. You may need to drink coffee without sugar 100 times before it tastes normal to you, but you absolutely can learn new habits. NEVER GIVE UP!
Tip #12	Get help when you need it. Medical help, counseling, a support group, spiritual guidance or a friend who has healthy habits for a positive role model. Don't hesitate to reach out for support. It's a rare person who can resist temptation alone.

I TRIED HYPNOSIS TO CONTROL MY CRAVINGS. IT WORKED TO REALLY WELL AND STRENGTHENED MY WILLPOWER.

In my decades of yoyo dieting and desperate attempts to lose weight and keep it off, I tried everything from private talk therapy to group talk therapy, doctor supervised diets, over-the-counter drugs and distraction tricks that I learned from friends, books and magazines.

But, hands down, the most effective way I've ever found to stop cravings is hypnosis.

Here's my family's experience: My mother was a chain-smoker for 40 years. She stopped cold after two hypnosis sessions. My aunt was a chain-smoker for +40 years. She stopped cold after three hypnosis session. I craved ice cream and all things cold and sweet. I lost my craving entirely after two hypnosis sessions. I craved pretzels and chips, loving the crunch and the salt. I lost my craving and was able to not be tempted at all after two hypnosis sessions.

The loss of craving lasted almost ten years for me before I needed to go back for a refresher session. My mother and aunt stopped smoking for life. My aunt is now nearly 90 and hasn't smoked for over 30 years.

The three of us went to three different hypno-therapists in three different parts of the country. Admittedly, this is a small statistical sample, but all three women in my family had similar experiences: Effective, complete relief for cravings, whether a physical addiction like my mother and aunt's addiction to nicotine, or mental temptation like my pull towards ice cream.

We supplemented the personal sessions with our licensed hypno-therapists by listening daily to tapes (or CDs) made to reinforce positive behavior to break negative habits. I listened to my recordings at bedtime, and often fell asleep to the soothing sound of the hypnotist's voice.

Go to a professional for private, 5-star treatment or buy a recording on Amazon

Going to a private professional will cost you about $150 a session. The fees vary, of course. A weekly session is suggested and this would not be unusual if you haven't done previous counseling about weight and eating issues. It could be very helpful for you. But, you can see that the money will really add up.

Going to a private professional hypno-therapist is the 5-star, white-glove, top-of-the-line way to do hypnosis for weight loss but it is expensive and you need to find an experienced practitioner in your area. If you live in a city, this shouldn't be a problem. If possible, check with a review service like www.Yelp.com for information on authenticated personal experiences.

If you're in a more rural area, consider buying weight related audios with pre-recorded sessions. You can find them on ITunes, Amazon and Audible.

I just searched on Amazon for "Hypnosis for weight loss" and found 194 results. Many of these look very promising. You can buy one for less than $10. Pick the recording that has the best reviews and appeals to you. Give it a try.

Hypnosis: How it works when you go to a professional hypno-therapist

A hypno-therapist who specializes in addictions and food cravings is most likely a trained and licensed psychotherapist who has learned hypnosis as a therapeutic tool. This is the kind of professional I would seek out if you have the resources.

It's possible you believe that hypnotists have a bad reputation as circus and stage performers and tricksters. I have been hypnotized on stage myself, and was shocked to find that the "tricks" actually worked on me. At the snap of a finger, I was crying like a baby or milking an imaginary cow.

Going to a hypo-therapist is nothing like this. I've been to three different hypno-therapists over the last 20 years and the experience with all three has been very similar. It starts out with a talk session, just like an introductory session with any therapist. They will ask about your goals, your fears and your challenges. If you are motivated to be helped, you will be open and co-operative. You may or may not be self-aware and be able to identify what is really driving you towards the desired food. The therapist may need to do some detective work and need additional sessions to identify the best way to help you. The reason my mother and I only needed two sessions to reveal what our core issues were is because both of us had done quite a lot of therapy already so we were able to give the hypno-therapist a jump-start.

The hypno-therapist will probably do a session on your first or second visit when you will be asked to lie down, relax and listen to suggestions. This is the hypnosis session. There will be about a 10-minute introduction with relaxing images, possibly of you walking on a beach. You will be asked to follow the hypnotist's suggested images and imagine yourself in the setting, doing what the hypnotist suggests. In my case, it was walking down the stairs to a beach, with every stair bringing me closer and closer to total relaxation. When I got to the sand, I was given gentle and positive suggestions and told positive ways to build my self-control.

Hypnosis is always positive.

You may be told to think about having a refreshing glass of water every time you think about having a soda. You will not be told that soda is bad. You will be given positive, active thoughts to replace the craving thoughts.

The hypnosis session lasts 30 to 60 minutes. You will not be tricked or asked to do anything foolish or threatening to your safety.

You can protect yourself further by choosing a hypno-therapist who practices in a professional building as part of a therapy group. I personally have never had a problem or any reason to feel unsafe or uncomfortable, nor have I heard of anyone having a problem.

Every once in a while, when I talk to someone new about being hypnotized, I hear about her fantasy that she's going to be unconscious on a couch and some unethical male hypnotist is going to rape her or take sexual advantage. Usually, this involves an image that she is in a nightgown and he is wearing a flowing black cape. This is really childish nonsense. If you are afraid of getting help because you think that fearful, unwanted sex will be involved, please consider that you may have more issues than just an unhealthy craving for sugar or ice cream. The solution is simple, anyway: go to a hypno-therapist who is a woman.

After your first or second visit, you will receive a recording of a one-hour hypnosis session custom made for you. You will be instructed to listen to it daily for a week, a month, or as long as needed. I have recordings that go back decades that I listen to occasionally for a refresher!

CDs and MP3 recordings for your IPod or smart phone make it easy

Your 30 to 60 minute hypnosis session is recorded. Your task is to listen it to daily to reinforce the positive suggestions, until they become ingrained behavior.

Sometimes, the hypnotist will record your custom session privately and have it ready for you on your next visit. This is how two of the three hypnotists I went to handled the recording. The third recorded our session live and handed me the recording. Today, hypno-therapists use the same kind of up-to-date MP3 and CD records that the rest of the world enjoys. You will be asked, however, what kind of technology you have available. If you don't have ANY way to play a recording, you will need to make this happen.

I prefer to receive CDs. I keep a CD player next to my bed and often listen while I fall asleep. Sometimes, I upload the recording to ITunes then put it on my IPhone so I can listen while I'm traveling.

Hypnosis works for cravings and general overeating

Let's suppose that you don't actually have cravings for specific foods but feel out of control about overeating in general. Let's imagine that you like to eat and chew and swallow everything in sight until you are stuffed.

Hypnosis can work for that, also. The urge to fill yourself is deep and complex. If you know that you are overeating, perhaps you have already given a lot of thought to "why am I doing this?" Self-medicating for sorrow, loneliness, sadness with overeating is a classic, tragic response to the troubles in our lives. You are not alone if you are an emotional eater. I did this for years. There's even a national support group which recognizes that overeating is commonplace and offers support: Overeaters Anonymous. https://oa.org This group has meetings face-to-face, online, on the telephone in both English and Spanish.

Please get the help you need. You don't need to go through resisting temptations alone!

Why don't diet professionals talk more about hypnosis?

You may wonder why—if hypnosis is so effective—it doesn't show up more on TV or in books and magazines as a weight control recommendation. Here are my thoughts about that:

- The best hypnosis is hypno-therapy with a licensed psychotherapist. It's awkward to say to a person who wants to lose weight "You need therapy". Can you imagine a magazine in a supermarket saying, "You're overeating so go to a shrink!"? Telling someone that they have issues is perilous for so many reasons. It's just easier to sell a new miracle diet.

- There is no financial reward recommending hypno-therapy for a talk-show host or magazine. Where is the product to sell? There's no book, no bottle of pills, no pre-made meals.

- Hypnosis puts the responsibility firmly on the individual's behavior. There is no escape to a magic pill or newly discovered fruit you can add to your diet to melt away fat. With hypnosis, it's all about you and the choices you are making. That's very uncomfortable for a lot of people who would rather find a quick cure.

Hypnosis can help you change unhealthy behaviors

If you are willing and ready, you will find professional hypnosis to be a very valuable tool. I did. Hypnosis therapy about overcoming my cravings has made my life so much easier. I highly recommend that you give it a try!

But, don't even think about amateur hypnotists. Your friend waving a watch back and forth across your face will not do anything except make you laugh, if it doesn't bore you first. As with any kind of therapy, find a trained professional to help you make a difference in your life.

A word about sugar: Sugar has addictive properties. Could you be hooked?

In *Habit #6: Avoid Added Sugars and Sweetened Drinks* we discussed the powerful effect that sugar has on your brain's functions. The human brain reacts to sugar like it reacts to a drug. Your brain and the metabolism it directs learn to depend on sugar, making it harder and harder to say "no".

Excess sugar in your bloodstream travels to the brain where it's the trigger to release dopamine, the powerful neurotransmitter that creates feelings of pleasure. With continued consumption of excess sugar, the brain develops a dependence on it to maintain dopamine levels. Then, when high levels of sugar aren't present in your bloodstream, as dopamine levels fall, you feel uncomfortable: moody, irritable, edgy and frustrated. This is the classic "sugar crash".

Grabbing foods with more sugar becomes an immediate priority.

So, if you are accustomed to eating sweetened foods and drinking soda or sweetened juices, stepping away from them permanently is going to be a challenge. Prepare yourself by learning as much as possible about the metabolic effects of sugar. (There are books about this in *Part Six: Resources for Learning More*. Plus, there is a wealth of information about sugar and health on the Internet.)

Realistically, reinventing your diet to minimize added sugar will be one of the most challenging things you will do. Be sure to check with your professional health care provider and get as much support as possible. Enlist your family members, ask a friend to be an "accountability buddy". Join a program such as Weight Watchers where you will find a group of motivated people with your same goal: to lose weight, keep it off and live a healthy lifestyle. In their weekly meetings you can discuss your challenges and learn how others are dealing with similar issues.

Whether progress is rapid or slow, don't lose faith that weight control is a longterm goal with longterm rewards. Finding support, encouragement and help will help you be strong today and believe that you can be stronger tomorrow. You can do this!

THE 4 WEEK PROGRAM TO LEARN THE 10 DAILY HABITS

**Shifting to a healthy lifestyle.
Here's how to start.**

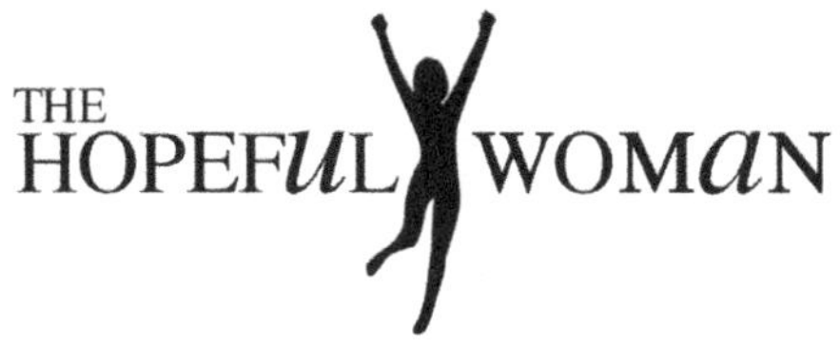

GETTING READY TO START

Time for action:
How to prepare to learn the
10 Daily Habits

This is your opportunity to learn new, healthy lifestyle habits!

One of the many reasons why weight loss diets don't work is because a diet is an intervention in your normal life. When you stop the program and go back to what you usually do, the pounds come back. So, the answer is obvious, isn't it? <u>You need to change your lifestyle</u>. You need to make your normal daily life support losing weight and keeping it off.

Many, if not all, of the 10 Daily Habits for Weight Control may be new to you, so trying to learn all of them at once could be overwhelming. For that reason, I'm suggesting a four-week program to begin living with the 10 Daily Habits.

The first week, you'll learn and practice only three new habits. The second week, you'll add only three more. In the third week, you'll learn the last four habits. By the fourth week, you will have experience with all 10 Daily Habits and the opportunity to absorb them over a month of practice.

Also, by week four, you'll know which habits are the most challenging for you so you can concentrate on practicing those while continuing to feel comfortable with the others.

Reinventing your lifestyle

Remember, the more you practice, the easier each habit becomes. It won't be long but you need to be realistic: there is a learning curve.

The key to success for any weight control habit is whether you can live with it for a long period of time. Practice and repetition are the only ways you can make new behaviors become normal, every day parts of life. And, unless you feel comfortable, you won't be able to sustain doing something month after month, year after year.

I'm living proof that the combination of these 10 Daily Habits work. I lost a total of 85 pounds and have kept them off comfortably. That bears repeating: *comfortably!* Friends who have met me during my Stable Period can't imagine that I used to struggle with my weight—they only know me as a trim and fit woman who enjoys eating, going to parties and out to restaurants.

It's all thanks to living with the 10 Daily Habits.

The transition period is the hardest part

Maintaining a weight control lifestyle is not hard…once you know how to do it. The hardest part—and this is true—is the transition period when you still want to do things your old way and the new behaviors still seem unusual. This will pass!

You may need help, in the form of a support group, counseling or a good friend to talk to and learn the 10 Daily Habits together. Going through a transition period is always more comfortable with a partner, at least for me. Overall, it's important to be realistic: choosing a lifestyle for weight control is a big, longterm commitment.

You are in this for life.

PREPARING FOR SUCCESS

If you were preparing to take a long trip, you would expect to spend some hours planning and packing for your journey. Preparing for a major lifestyle change is no different. You should expect to spend some time getting ready.

If you haven't done these steps to prepare, the time is now.

Step #1: Check with your doctor

As with the start of any program that focuses on your overall health, you should check with your medical doctor. You should have your blood pressure, blood cholesterol and blood sugar levels checked. Please bring a copy of the 10 Daily Habits and discuss them with your doctor to make sure that they will be appropriate for your personal situation.

Step #2: Inform the people who share your home about your commitment to lifestyle changes

If you live with family members or roommates, review how you will be changing your eating and sleeping habits. And why. It's your commitment to your longterm health. If you have a spouse, hopefully you can learn the 10 Daily Habits together and help reinforce each other's commitment to a healthy lifestyle. If you are worried about being sabotaged or having your new choices questioned or attacked, please seek help from a support group or health professional.

Step #3: Review your food sources

Consider where you currently buy food and meals and think about whether food from those retailers will support your healthy choices. If not, you'll need to research new food outlets. If you are lucky to have a farmer's market, Trader Joes, Costco, Whole Foods or independent health food stores near you, take a walk through and locate the whole grains.

Be aware that finding substitutes for refined white flour will be one of your greatest challenges. The stuff is simply everywhere. Fortunately, more and more people are waking up to how dangerous refined white flour is to our health and demanding more whole grain products at food markets, fast food outlets and restaurants.

Step #4: Be good to yourself

Be kind and patient with yourself. It took me 5 years to find and internalize these 10 Daily Habits. You've jumped past the time spent discovering and experimenting by reading this book, but you still need to practice,

practice, practice. There is no substitute for continued repetition to make sustained, permanent changes in your eating and lifestyle habits.

Be patient! Have faith! YOU CAN DO THIS!

THE 10 DAILY HABITS
WEEKLY WORKSHEET

70 Opportunities to get it right

Keep track of your progress with this weekly worksheet. (You can download unlimited free copies on www.HopefulWoman.com.) Documenting your daily progress is powerful. As you stay on task, you'll feel tremendous pride as your worksheets fill up. And, you'll be practicing your new habits for weight control.

Every day, as you're getting ready for bed, check off which habit you've been able to practice successfully that day at least once. Post this worksheet in your bathroom where you will see it first thing in the morning to be reminded, and last thing at night to review your day. You could also carry a copy in your purse.

If you have been challenged by practicing any habit, go back to that chapter and review.

There are 70 boxes to check off on this worksheet every week. That's a lot to accomplish! Celebrate the habits you've been able to master and renew your commitment to the habits, which still need extra focus.

Try to increase the numbers of your checked boxes every week.

Celebrate your success! If you can steadily increase the boxes checked, you are doing wonderfully well.

Be proud of your steady progress!

10 DAILY HABITS WEEKLY WORKSHEET

	Mon	Tues	Wed	Thurs	Fri	Sat	Sun
Habit #1: Get enough sleep	Hours	Hours	Hours	Hours	Hours	Hours	Hours
Habit #2: Start the day well with a breakfast of protein and whole grains							
Habit #3: Exercise for 30 minutes every day	Minutes	Minutes	Minutes	Minutes	Minutes	Minutes	Minutes
Habit #4: Learn and practice portion Control							
Habit #5: Know what's in the food you eat							
Habit #6: Avoid added sugars & sweetened drinks							
Habit #7: Find substitutes for refined white flour							
Habit #8: Snack often							
Habit #9: Enjoy at least one non-caloric pleasure every day							
Habit #10: Control your food cravings							
WEEKLY TOTALS:							

Available as a PDF for free download at: www.HopefulWoman.com

Notes:

WEEK ONE: PRACTICE THESE 3 DAILY HABITS FIRST

Start the first week with three habits that focus on sleep, breakfast and exercise. You already do at least two of these, so adjustments for a weight control lifestyle will be easy to understand. There are habits coming up in the following weeks that will require research and more thought, but let's make the first week easy so you can get used to thinking about weight control and shifting your lifestyle as you go through your day.

- Habit #1: Get enough sleep.

- Habit #2: Start the day well with breakfast.

- Habit #3: Exercise for 30 minutes every day

Be sure to thoroughly read the chapters covering each habit in detail so you understand why they are important to learn and sustain.

HABIT #1: GET ENOUGH SLEEP

Willpower and appetite are affected by lack of sleep. Getting enough sleep is a must for taking off pounds and controlling your weight.

DETAILS: Pages 39 to 53

PREPARATION: The time and effort you invest in improving your sleep habits will yield you life-long benefits. Most people need between 7 and 8 hours.

Here are suggestions to improve your bedtime preparations and quality of your sleep.

- Do the best you can to make your bedroom "sleep friendly". If it's noisy, buy earplugs or a white noise machine. (I sleep with earplugs every night. Now, my brain is programmed to know that when the plugs go in, it settles down to sleep.)

- If your bed is uncomfortable, change it if you can. Sometimes, a foam topper works miracles.

- Commit to using your bed only for sleep. Answer emails somewhere else.

- Spend time on bedtime rituals. If you can, don't rush. Stretch them out to give yourself time to unwind.

- Don't drink coffee late in the day.

- Don't drink alcohol just before going to bed.

- Allow at least three hours between exercising and bedtime.

- If you can, set regular bedtimes and waking times.

- Turn off the TV. Don't fall asleep with the TV or radio still on. The sound will stimulate your brain and interfere with the depth of your sleep.

- Achieving orgasm is a great soporific. (Sleep aid.)

- If you have a bad back, hip or neck problems, experiment with extra pillows to make yourself comfortable. Target sells pillows very inexpensively if you need more.

- If you think you have a sleep disorder, be sure to consult with your doctor.

- If you have sleep apnea, or suspect that you do, don't hesitate to get medical help.

HABIT #2:
START THE DAY WELL WITH BREAKFAST

Eat protein and whole grains to jump-start your metabolism. Do not eat added sugars! Read all labels on breakfast "foods". If you have protein and whole grains with plenty of fiber, not only will you feel better throughout the morning, you will also inspire confidence in yourself by launching the day with good habits. Start well, stay well!

DETAILS: Pages 55 to 80

PREPARATION: Keep a week's supply of healthy breakfast materials on hand in your kitchen. I recommend disposing of all the junk cereals, crackers and chips in your home.

Remember, "whole wheat" is not "whole grain". There are many different types of grains to try: oats, millet, brown rice, spelt.

Generally, I like to have breakfast foods in my kitchen that will have an extended shelf life. The exception, of course, is soft fresh fruit, but basics like whole grain cereal, apples, eggs, yogurt and milk will certainly last a week or more.

Whenever possible, buy organic products.

Here's what to stock in your kitchen for breakfasts:

- Fresh eggs: boil 50% for quick morning protein.

- Whole grain hot cereal: oatmeal, multi-grain.

- Whole grain cold cereal: read the labels carefully before you buy.

- Whole grain bread. Can be frozen and used one slice at a time.

- Rice cakes.

- Milk, soymilk or almond milk. Read the label to avoid added sugars. Buy the unsweetened variety.

- Fresh oranges, melon or fruit. (No juice! Processed juice is not your friend. If you juice your own fruit and vegetables, OK, but it's better to eat the whole fruit or vegetable.)

- Butter or butter substitute for cooking the eggs.

- Optional: roasted chicken for protein. (I often have a market rotisserie chicken on hand as part of my quick breakfast.)

- Optional: plain, whole milk yogurt for topping your cereal.

- Optional: Peanut or nut butter for a quick spread to go.

HABIT #3:
EXERCISE 30 MINUTES EVERY DAY

Teach yourself that a day without exercise is a day that's incomplete. Learn to fidget.

Exercise is the "magic bullet" we've all been looking for to improve our health. You can start at any age. And, moving your body is free! Fidgeting is an underappreciated way to keep your muscles moving. Flex, squeeze, rotate, twist—you can fidget anytime, anywhere.

DETAILS: Pages 81 to 92

PREPARATION: If you are not exercising at all now, a doctor's OK is a must before you start any exercise program.

- An exercise buddy will make it easier to get started and stick with a regular program. Look around for a friend or colleague who can be your fitness partner.

- Learning to fidget is healthier than sitting still at your desk. Fight the urge to be sedentary!

- Buy a pedometer. Whether you plan to making walking your primary exercise or not, studies have shown that monitoring the number of steps you take daily is a big motivator for more movement.

- Review your daily schedule and be realistic where and how you can get at least 30 minutes of exercise every day.

- Check to see if your employer offers a fitness program or workout facilities.

- Group exercise programs can be very enjoyable and easy to stick with. Don't be self-conscious about joining an exercise class. You will find people of all body sizes.

- Most communities have a variety of health clubs and fitness centers at different price levels. The YMCA is a wonderful resource for fitness options if you have one near you. Community centers offer classes without a membership requirement.

- Some people have success with DVDs at home. You can read reviews and chose exercise DVDs on Amazon. For years, when

I was too busy to get to a gym regularly, I practiced yoga at home by following a DVD. For cardio exercise, I used my home treadmill. (Surveys reveal that of all the home exercise equipment available, the treadmill has the best record for people using it consistently.)

- Before you go to sleep at night, plan your time for exercise the next day.

WEEK ONE: DAILY HABITS WORKSHEET

	Mon	Tues	Wed	Thurs	Fri	Sat	Sun
Habit #1: Get enough sleep	Hours	Hours	Hours	Hours	Hours	Hours	Hours
Habit #2: Start the day well with a breakfast of protein and whole grains							
Habit #3: Exercise for 30 minutes every day	Minutes	Minutes	Minutes	Minutes	Minutes	Minutes	Minutes
WEEKLY TOTALS:							

Was I pleased with my success?

	Mon	Tues	Wed	Thurs	Fri	Sat	Sun
Yes! I really applied what I learned about weight control and good health. GREAT JOB!							
Well, I had challenges. Tomorrow I can do better. I will do better.							

Where can I use improvement?

Which actions am I going to take next week?

Notes:

WEEK TWO:
ADD THE NEXT 3 DAILY HABITS

Add three more daily habits to your lifestyle this week. These habits focus on your relationship with food.

- Habit #4: Learn and practice portion control

- Habit #5: Know what's in your food before you put it in your mouth.

- Habit #6: Avoid added sugars and sweetened drinks.

These are complicated subjects that are key to mastering weight control. Be patient and expect that controlling your portions and most importantly, knowing what's in your food, will be life-long goals.

Go back and review the chapters covering each habit in detail so you understand why they are important. Take notes when you need to, or carry this book with you during the day for a quick refresher.

Are you overwhelmed? You can always slow down the pace and add a new habit to practice only after you have mastered the previous one. Most people would not want to wait 10 weeks to learn 10 Daily Habits, but there is nothing wrong in taking on only one habit each week. Feel free to go at your own pace.

And remember: mastery takes practice, practice, practice!

HABIT #4:
LEARN & PRACTICE PORTION CONTROL

Keep your body running smoothly and comfortably all day long. Pay special attention to not letting your blood sugar level drop so you aren't extra-hungry and want to grab any food you can, or overeat.

DETAILS: Pages 93 to 108

PREPARATION: This habit requires paying strong attention with your eyes and training yourself to what the size of portions look like.

- If you don't own a measuring cup and spoons, buy them now.

- Practice measuring out cupfuls of different foods (cereals, raisins, rice, milk, water, yogurt, ice cream – anything you have) and putting them on plates or in bowls and glasses. Take a good look at how much volume is actually in a cupful.

- Do the same with the tablespoon measure.

- If you have a kitchen or postal scale, measure one ounce of cheese so you can memorize the volume. Measure out three ounces of chicken or fish and study what it looks like on a plate. You can also hold the cheese and chicken in the palm of your hand to get a good sense of what a normal, three ounce portion of meat looks like.

- Assess the plates, bowls, cups and glasses you usually eat from and consider replacing them with smaller sizes.

- Invest $10 in small plastic storage containers so you can measure take-out into smaller portions.

You only need to measure your foods once. Try to memorize what the volume looks like visually. You will find this recognition skill very helpful, especially at restaurants.

HABIT #5:
KNOW WHAT'S IN YOUR FOOD
BEFORE YOU PUT IT IN YOUR MOUTH

Read labels. Learn about calories, carbohydrates, fats and fiber. To lose weight and KEEP IT OFF you really need to know what you're eating. Being aware of what's in the food and how it affects your body is critical for lifelong weight control.

The human digestive system and how it works is a dynamic field of scientific research with new discoveries all the time. It's a fascinating topic! I sincerely hope that reading this book inspires you to be curious and want to learn more.

Here's a popular saying: "Food is either slow medicine or slow poison." Be aware of what you're eating and do your very best to make healthy choices.

DETAILS: Pages 109 to 136

PREPARATION: Understanding how the ingredients in your food affect your metabolism is a life skill. If this is new to you, be prepared that there is a lot to learn! It's absolutely worth every minute to be able to protect your health.

- Buy a handy pocket guide to calories, carbohydrates and fats. They are often for sale at hospital pharmacies or at checkout counters in supermarkets. Or, there are similar apps available for your smart phone.

- Writing down what you eat is very helpful. Buy a pocket notebook, an actual food diary or find an app to keep track of what you're eating every day. Studies have shown that people who keep food diaries lose twice as much weight as people who don't! (See *Bonus Habit #2: Keep a Food Diary.*)

- Commit to reading every label before you buy any packaged food.

HABIT #6:
AVOID ADDED SUGARS & SWEETENED DRINKS

Understand sucrose, glucose and fructose and what turns on your brain's Pleasure Center. Be alert to sugars hiding in your food. You can move past wanting sugar!

It's especially important that you learn as much as possible about how your body metabolizes sugar. Please read the full chapter *Habit #6: Avoid Added Sugars and Sweetened Drinks.* You will have a better understanding about why sugar is so dangerous for anyone trying to control their weight.

DETAILS: Pages 137 to 154

PREPARATION: Learn as much as you possibly can about sugar's unhealthy effects on your body and commit proactively to wean yourself off sugar and added sweeteners.

- Identify sweetened products in your kitchen and eliminate any that are snacks, breakfast cereals, sweetened yogurts, sodas and sweetened juices. A package of sugar for baking is OK to keep. (Let's assume that you don't bake mounds of sweet foods very often.)

- Commit to not bringing sweetened products into your home or office.

- Buy and prepare your substitute go-to items when you have a sugar craving: gum, fresh vegetables to crunch, raisins to suck on, small portion of whole grain cereal. Gum really works for me.

- Set yourself a forgiving timeline to adjust your tastes. Example: It simply takes a while to learn to like coffee without sugar. You can do it!

- Remember: 15 Tasting tries are needed—at least—to shift your preferences.

WEEK TWO: DAILY HABITS WORKSHEET

	Mon	Tues	Wed	Thurs	Fri	Sat	Sun
Habit #1: Get enough sleep	Hours	Hours	Hours	Hours	Hours	Hours	Hours
Habit #2: Start the day well with a breakfast of protein and whole grains							
Habit #3: Exercise for 30 minutes every day	Minutes	Minutes	Minutes	Minutes	Minutes	Minutes	Minutes
Habit #4: Learn and practice portion control							
Habit #5: Know what's in the food you eat							
Habit #6: Avoid added sugars & sweetened drinks							
WEEKLY TOTALS:							

Was I pleased with my success?

	Mon	Tues	Wed	Thurs	Fri	Sat	Sun
Yes! I really applied what I learned about weight control and good health. GREAT JOB!							
Well, I had challenges. Tomorrow I can do better. I will do better.							

Where can I use improvement?

Which actions am I going to take next week?

Notes:

WEEK THREE:
ADD 4 MORE DAILY HABITS
& YOU'VE TRIED THEM ALL

Week Three is the most challenging. Here's why: you are still practicing the first six Daily Habits and now there are four more to learn.

- Habit #7: Find substitutes for refined white flour

- Habit #8: Snack often

- Habit #9: Enjoy at least one non-caloric pleasure every day

- Habit #10: Learn to control your food cravings

It helps to remember that weight control is a lifelong commitment. As long as you maintain your commitment to take off weight and keep it off, and you continue to practice integrating these habits into your daily life, you will make progress. Shifting behaviors and forming new habits takes time and practice.

What about all those quick diets that promise it's going to be easy? Well, they lied. That's one of the reasons their diets don't work to keep your weight off. It's not easy.

Weight control is a complex skill that requires paying attention and repetition, just like any other life skill. But, the good news is that humans are very adaptable. You will be amazed at how soon you can shift to a healthier lifestyle. You can do this!

HABIT #7:
FIND SUBSTITUTES FOR REFINED WHITE FLOUR

Eat whole grains. Be willing to try new grains and choose the healthiest substitutes you can afford. Learn how refined white flour metabolizes dangerously fast and why you should avoid it.

DETAILS: Pages 155 to 170

PREPARATION: It will always be a benefit to you if you broaden the selection of foods that you're willing to eat because you'll have more choices. We all have favorite foods, especially those we learned to love in childhood. But, maybe they aren't doing our older bodies any good. Avoiding refined white flour is a major step in moving towards a healthy lifestyle to control your weight.

- Read and understand the difference between "whole wheat" and "whole grain". See the chapter on *Habit #6: Find Substitutes for Refined White Flour*.

- Walk through your neighborhood food store looking for whole grain products. Talk to the manager about stocking more.

- Research other markets in your neighborhood.

- Clear out room in your freezer so you can freeze whole grain breads.

- Clear out room in your cabinet so you can store dry whole grains as ready-to-eat cereals or grains to cook.

- Buy storage containers for buying whole grains in bulk at Whole Foods and other markets.

- Talk to your family about how refined white flour is metabolized and why it's healthier to find other grains to eat.

HABIT #8:
SNACK OFTEN

Plan ahead to avoid junk food. Say "NO" to empty calories.

DETAILS: Pages 171 to 183

PREPARATION: It's important to avoid sugar and sweetened drinks for your snacks. Choose a small portion of a high-fiber food that will take some time to digest so your blood sugar stays level and doesn't drop quickly.

- Invest in small plastic containers and baggies to be ready to carry healthy snacks with you.

- Buying healthy snack foods (nuts, vegetables, yogurt without sugar) in larger quantities will save you money. Use your own containers to divide them into snack-size portions.

- Make a commitment every morning as you brush your teeth that you are not going to snack mindlessly. You will make deliberate decisions about everything that passes into your mouth.

- Stock a week of snacks in your kitchen or office. Don't be caught with nothing when your blood sugar starts to drop.

- Repeat successful snacks day after day. You don't have to eat something new if there is a healthy snack that you really like. Choose it again and again.

Don't skip meals!

This is very important. Depriving your body of food and your brain of its energy source will backfire on you. Your blood sugar will crash and you'll be vulnerable to eating impulsively, grabbing whatever is in front of you, which, in this day and age, is probably fast food filled with fat, sugar and refined white flour.

Repeating the same snacks works for me

Once I've found something that tastes good, is full of fiber and makes me feel good, I don't mind snacking on the same food every day. My favorites are sliced apples and a handful of almonds. If I'm craving something sweet, my go-to snack is raisins.

HABIT #9:
ENJOY AT LEAST ONE NON-CALORIC PLEASURE EVERY DAY

Stimulate all your senses: Touch, smell, sight, hearing, taste. Enjoy your body: Have more orgasms!

DETAILS: Pages 185 to 195

PREPARATION: How could this not be the most enjoyable of all the 10 Habits! Prepare to make yourself feel good and keep feeling good.

- Consider what activities or sensations not involving food/drink have given you the most pleasure. Make the longest list you can. It could include simple items like feeling a soft fabric, petting your cat, watching a sunset or smelling a lovely candle. It could also include extravagant items like the wind in your hair while on a balloon ride. Review the list often to reinforce that you deserve pleasure.

- Be alert to opportunities for non-caloric pleasures as you go through your day. Did your morning shampoo smell wonderful, and, if not, can you get yourself a shampoo you love? Did you enjoy the warm water in your shower running between your legs? Was there a beautiful voice on your car's radio? Did your children smile and hug you? Did you notice any good smells or new textures? If you're interested in music, treat yourself to new downloads or CDs for music that makes you happy.

- More orgasms should be on every person's weight control agenda. If you need privacy, look for time in your day when you can give that to yourself. If your sex life involves a partner, enjoy knowing together that orgasms are a key element in overall physical fitness.

- Confirm that you have any supplies that you need to achieve orgasm comfortably. If you would benefit from a lubricant, you can find a wide variety on Amazon. If you need a vibrator or think a new one with a different design would perk up your sex life, now's the time to get yourself what you need.

- Buy new underpants. Bright colors, wild patterns are good. Reinforce your commitment to weight control and your physical pleasure every time you see them.

- If you can afford it, put new linens on your bed as a way of reinforcing the new era.

HABIT #10:
LEARN TO CONTROL YOUR FOOD CRAVINGS

Learn to deal with excessive desire and get help when you need it.

DETAILS: Pages 197 to 215

PREPARATION: This habit may require additional research and professional help. My own cravings required the help of a hypnotist to control.

- Make a realistic assessment of which foods and drinks call to you.

- If you have sugar cravings, please talk to your doctor.

- If you have alcohol cravings, please talk to a professional.

- For other, less serious cravings, review the chapter on how to distract your brain.

- Learn to be aware of your food environment. If you crave unhealthy foods with empty calories, don't buy them! Don't make excuses that you're buying them for your family because they want them. Nobody needs empty calories.

- Planning ahead to avoid temptation is always a better strategy than trying to talk yourself out of a craving once its heat is upon you.

WEEK THREE: DAILY HABITS WORKSHEET

	Mon	Tues	Wed	Thurs	Fri	Sat	Sun
Habit #1: Get enough sleep	Hours	Hours	Hours	Hours	Hours	Hours	Hours
Habit #2: Start the day well with a breakfast of protein and whole grains							
Habit #3: Exercise for 30 minutes every day	Minutes	Minutes	Minutes	Minutes	Minutes	Minutes	Minutes

Habit #4: Learn and practice portion control							
Habit #5: Know what's in the food you eat							
Habit #6: Avoid added sugars & sweetened drinks							
Habit #7: Find substitutes for refined white flour							
Habit #8: Snack often							
Habit #9 Enjoy at least one non-caloric pleasure every day							
Habit #10: Control your food cravings							
WEEKLY TOTALS:							

Was I pleased with my success?

	Mon	Tues	Wed	Thurs	Fri	Sat	Sun
Yes! I really applied what I learned about weight control and good health. GREAT JOB!							
Well, I had challenges. Tomorrow I can do better. I will do better.							

Where can I use improvement?

Which actions am I going to take next week?

Notes:

WEEK FOUR:
PUTTING IT ALL TOGETHER
AS YOUR LIFESTYLE

Congratulations! You've completed three weeks of weight control practice. And, if you've followed the program, you have probably lost several pounds as well. In future weeks, you will lose more weight, slowly and steadily.

And now, it's time to be realistic and review how you're doing.

Having trouble practicing or sustaining any of the 10 Daily Habits?

By now, you should be aware which habits are giving you the most challenges.

While all of the 10 Daily Habits are easy to learn, they are not equally easy to put into practice in your daily life. You may have instant success with *Habit #4: Learn and Practice Portion Control* but struggle to make a daily practice of *Habit #7: Find Substitutes for Refined White Flour.*

What to do if you're having trouble? First, go back and study each challenging habit and make sure you really understand the health benefits. Look closely at all the tips offered for making changes. Then, focus on feeling comfortable with your knowledge.

Consider slowing down and taking the time to practice one single habit at your own pace instead of three or four at a time. Mastering one habit each week may be the best tactic for you. Don't worry if you need to add extra weeks. It's not a race—this is the rest of your life! Take your time to really internalize new behaviors.

The most important thing is to keep trying every single day, and know that these habits put together will really control your weight.

Making lifestyle changes takes patience and practice, but you can absolutely learn to adapt to new habits

Humans are adaptable. We are hard-wired to learn new things. There is no other species on the planet that can change like we can! We've gone from caves to the moon because we were willing to try and learn new things. You do not need to be stuck. You can free yourself from a lifetime of yo-yo dieting by being willing to practice new habits.

Stick with it. You will soon be surprised at how adaptable you are.

We're all impatient, especially to lose that extra weight, but it helps to accept that longterm weight control is not a quick fix. Patience and practice are your keys to absorbing the new habits that will control your weight. That's just the way it is. As you know from a lifetime of losing and gaining weight, there is no magic bullet. Practice and patience is what works. There is no escaping that learning new habits will take time and repetition.

But here's where the gift of human adaptability comes in: The more you practice, the easier each habit gets. You can absolutely do this!

Use the 10 Daily Habits Weekly Worksheet

The 10 Habit Weekly Worksheet will give you visual confirmation of which habits are easy for you to absorb and which are giving you daily challenges. This is especially helpful information.

By marking off which habits you've been able to practice that day, soon you'll have tangible evidence of how you're successfully mastering a weight control lifestyle. And, you will also see clearly which habits are stumbling blocks for you so you can refocus your effort wisely, where it's most needed.

Success is more than numbers on your scale! Checking off the habits you've been practicing is a great way to feel encouraged and stay motivated. You can applaud yourself for successfully putting each habit into practice.

Get help and support if you need it

Most of us need help and support and it comes in many different forms. I didn't have one steady, constant source of support, throughout the years, but dipped in and out of many different types. From a friend, to organized weight-loss groups, to a hypnosis therapist, to personal counseling, to nutrition classes, I have sought out the help and support from people whose profession is to focus on good health.

Don't be shy about asking for help. In my life, two of the most powerful sentences on my weight control journey have been *"Can you help me?"* and *"Will you teach me?"*

There are two ways of looking at support: external and internal. External support provides structure, a leader or group to join and a regular schedule. Internal support is entirely up to you. Personally, I find that external support has been far more effective in keeping me on track with weight control.

What kind of support available for you is determined by your motivation and your budget. Most of us can't afford to go to a private counselor or hire a personal trainer, but, fortunately, there are many low-cost alternatives available.

Having a weekly appointment will help keep you on track

Going for professional counseling every week is the gold standard for help staying on track with your weight goals. This is an expensive option, however. If your doctor recommends that you lose weight, please check with your health insurance carrier as, perhaps, professional help is covered.

There are a lot of other options that are not expensive. Weight Watchers is a weekly support group that is very helpful. They have their own weight loss programs, but I found the company of other people who want to take off extra pounds and keep them off to be motivating.

It helped me to have the structure of a weekly meeting. Although I didn't follow the specific Weight Watcher program, I appreciated their commitment. Plus, locations of weekly meetings are easy to find, and the cost was usually under $10. Casual conversations with other attendees can lead to supportive friendships for you, as it did for me.

Many community health centers offer nutrition classes that are helpful. And, it's a good way to meet your neighbors who have the same goals. Gyms and health clubs also offer classes, or their staff would be able to recommend where you could go. If you are a Kaiser Permanente member, they offer a range of free classes on weight and nutrition, plus a wide variety of online materials.

There are online support groups and communities you can sign up for. I like www.sparkpeople.com because their focus is longterm weight loss and maintaining a healthy weight. I don't agree with all of their suggestions about foods that are good to eat, (like refined white flour/pasta which I avoid), but their site is filled with other useful suggestions.

When you sign up for an online community, you receive email notices in your inbox daily. Even if you don't open them, just being reminded is useful because it helps reinforce your identity as someone who is taking control of your weight situation and doing something about it.

Finding a partner or 'accountability buddy'

It's great to have a cheerleader and someone who understands the details of your changes and challenges. Could this be a family member? Or, your best friend? Open a discussion about which habits are hardest for you to adopt and ask for their help.

Sometimes, it's helpful to start fresh, with a new person. Be on the lookout for someone who could be a new friend and confidant.

Increase your confidence by sharing your knowledge

Once your weight loss starts showing, you'll be amazed by the number of people who are curious about how you're doing it. That's the time to share what you've been learning.

There's nothing like teaching to strengthen your own knowledge of the subject. Plus, it feels really great to be able to help other people improve their health as you are working towards your own healthy lifestyle.

Be empowered. Remind yourself often that "You can do this!"

Don't forget that you can be proactive about encouraging yourself. Anything you can do to reinforce your identity as someone who is in control, and can take good care of her body, will help you stay focused on your goal of weight control.

If you actively look for ways to encourage and support yourself, everyday life will offer you opportunities that you might not expect.

Here are a few things I've done to remind myself that "*You can do this!*":

- Plan and have breakfast ready each morning so I am confident about starting the day with a good habit and good foundation for healthy living.

- Gather up and display visual reminders about weight control. Some people write empowering notes to themselves and post them around the house. One of my friends has a "wish board" in her closet with pictures of beautiful clothes she'd like to be able to wear. Another friend has a picture of a beach on his desk to remind him of running down the beach, being active and athletic.

- Sign up for nutrition and healthy living email newsletters. When I check my email, and see emails focusing on healthy living, it reminds me and reinforces my commitment. If I have time, I read them. If not, I am still reminded to stay focused that day. Receiving a steady stream of newsletters also reinforces that I am someone who values continuing education. It strengthens my resolve to learn as much as I can to take good care of myself. (See *Part Five: Resources* for recommendations.

- Collect a library of books on nutrition and display them at home. In my bathroom, I also leave books and magazines about healthy lifestyles. Guess what gets read during "private time"!

- Clear my home and personal workspace of short-term temptations. See no evil! But I keep a fruit bowl in my kitchen at all times. When I see fruit, it reminds me that I don't need to eat sweets and processed foods.

- Keep an exercise bag in my car where I can see it, ready to go. I am reminded that I can exercise and I'm ready. The bag contains athletic shoes and socks, a sports bra, leggings, a teeshirt, and a water bottle. I also keep a hiking stick in my car, so if the opportunity comes up to·go for a walk with friend, I am ready. Whenever I open my car door, I see the gym bag and am reminded that I can do it!

- Weigh myself only once a week, at most. My focus is on daily habits, not a daily number on the scale.

There are many more tips throughout all chapters on the 10 Daily Habits on how you can stay motivated. For specific tips about avoiding temptation, see *Habit #10: Control Your Food Cravings.*

PART FOUR:

BONUS HABITS

**Four more useful habits
which will help you develop a healthy lifestyle
and control your weight**

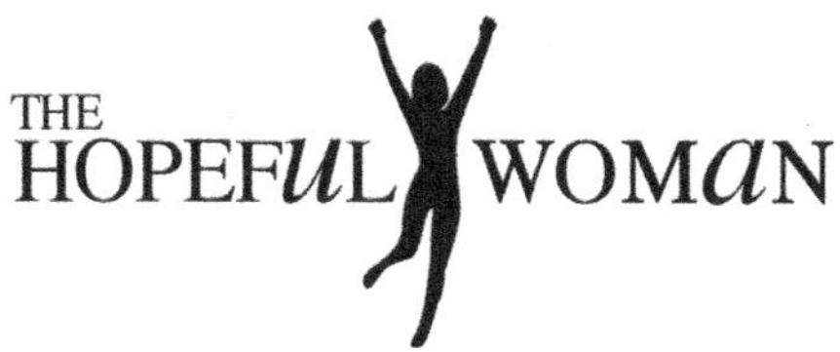

BONUS HABIT #1
READ ALL INGREDIENT &
NUTRITION LABELS.
IGNORE SALES SLOGANS

If the food has a nutrition or ingredient label,
never put it in your mouth until you've read everything.

Wouldn't it be a perfect world if we could trust all of our food suppliers to know about good nutrition and put our well being ahead of their profit margins? We could just buy any box of processed foods without a worry or extra thought. In this perfect world, all ingredients would be wholesome and support our good health. We would never have to be suspicious about additives, chemicals or hidden sugars. We could just relax and eat.

I wish it were that way—it sounds like the Garden of Eden. Sadly, that's not where we find ourselves as consumers in today's food chain.

These days, most of us live in cities, which nutritionist classify as "food deserts". That's right. This horrible term, "food deserts", is an accurate description for our environment, which requires all food and water to be brought in from the outside. Our cities are decorative, barren landscapes, so when we are out "hunting and gathering" for food, everything we find is the result of choices other people have made for us and delivered to our cities.

Everyone wants to be paid for their work or investments, and companies that produce food are no different. There has to be enough profit in the selling price to pay for the ingredients, the people who grew and prepared it, the people who work to transport and distribute the food, and the companies that sell it to you. And the stockholders who invest in the whole process. That's a lot of financial burden for a box of breakfast cereal.

Processed foods are not just foods. They're manufactured products.

You have no control over what goes into these products (except when our government steps in to remove dangerous ingredients). The only control you have is whether you are going to put these products in your mouth.

I say "Learn about what you eat first. Think about whether it's a healthy choice for you BEFORE you buy and eat them."

You must be your best advocate for your health.

For weight control, it is simply a requirement that you read all labels and do your best to decipher them. This is not always easy. Food manufacturers don't make it simple for you. Boxes are covered with marketing slogans that proclaim goodness. But, in the USA, packaged foods must have nutrition labels. If you are serious about controlling your weight, you must get in the habit of reading them before you buy any packaged food.

It's always wise to read labels. Here's how.

This is a sample nutrition label for macaroni and cheese. You can find it, along with very useful information on the Food and Drug Administration website: *How to Understand and Use the Nutrition Facts Label*. Since the FDA regulates nutrition labels, I thought it would be good to go right to the source for information. www.fda.gov/Food/IngredientsPackagingLabeling/LabelingNutrition.

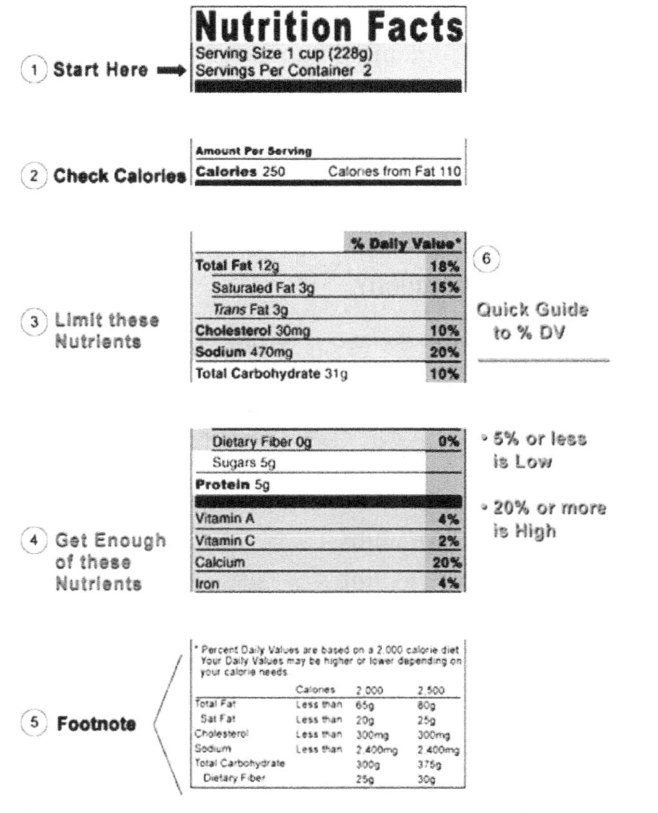

1. Start here:

Let's start with portion control. One of the easiest ways to get confused about labels is to think

that the package is the whole portion, especially if you're checking calories. Be sure to check "Servings per container". Don't forget that the number of servings you eat will determine how many calories you're consuming.

2. Calories:

Calories are the measure of how much energy you get from eating this food. The energy actually

comes from glucose, when your digestive system breaks the food down.

Calories from fat are another matter entirely because there is little or no possibility of the fat containing nutrients you need. Sure, you need omega 3s and linoleic acid but it doesn't take very much fish oil or vegetable oil to provide this. It certainly doesn't require eating food whose calories are 44% fat. Those fat calories are not beneficial to you and will damage your efforts at weight control.

3. and 4. Nutrients. How much?

Many studies show that the average adult should eat 2,000 calories daily to remain healthy, and this is the agreed standard by the FDA. The percentage of daily value of fat, cholesterol, carbohydrates, vitamins, etc., is based on eating that amount. (It's worth noting that the numbers on nutrition labels are something of a moving target and are frequently revised by the FDA as more is learned about health and nutrition.)

	% Daily Value*
Total Fat 12g	18%
Saturated Fat 3g	15%
Trans Fat 3g	
Cholesterol 30mg	10%
Sodium 470mg	20%
Total Carbohydrate 31g	10%

Dietary Fiber 0g	0%
Sugars 5g	
Protein 5g	
Vitamin A	4%
Vitamin C	2%
Calcium	20%
Iron	4%

For weight control purposes there are four primary numbers on labels you should pay attention to:

- Calories per serving

- Calories from fat. (Memorize that 1 gram of fat = 9 calories.)

- Grams of sugar. (Memorize that 1 gram of sugar = 4 calories.)

- Grams of protein. (Memorize that 1 gram of protein = 4 calories.)

Labels may surprise you with how much sugar is in packaged foods! Read low-fat labels especially carefully.

As discussed in previous chapters, you can live and thrive not eating a morsel of sugar. The amount of dietary fat we actually need to stay healthy is very small. And some of us have been advised to cut down on our salt intake.

When the low-fat craze hit in the 1970's, food manufacturers replaced the flavor from fat with sugar. When you are trying to avoid added sugars and sweeteners, you must be vigilant about reading the labels on low-fat or fat-free foods.

Here's an example: Wishbone Fat Free Ranch Dressing gets 40% of its calories from sugar. Here's the calculation from their nutrition label:

Total calories in 2 tablespoons:	30 calories
Total grams of sugar:	3 grams
Sugar is 4 calories per gram:	4 calories x 3 grams = 12 calories
Find the percentage:	12 ÷ 30 = .40 = 40%

For more instructions on how to calculate percentages, see *Habit #5: Know What's in Your Food.* It does get much, much easier with practice.

You need to read the labels for breakfast foods very carefully, also. You'll see sugar or a sweetener like corn syrup listed right up at the top of the ingredients. It's shocking, actually, how many packaged breakfast foods are loaded with sugar, including most boxed cereals, breakfast bars and pastries. For all your meals during the day, it's most important that you don't have a breakfast full of sugar. Fortunately, breakfast can be an easy meal with eggs, oatmeal or other whole grain, unsweetened cereals.

Is reading labels tiresome? Sorry. You can't control your weight without making this a habit. Don't want to do it? Just eat whole foods!

If you want to control your weight, there is no escaping the need to know what's in your food. You must develop the habit of reading all nutrition labels on packaged foods, and most importantly, understanding what the names and numbers mean.

Is it a pain to have to do this when you're shopping for food? Yes. Do it anyway.

The only time you can skip reading labels is if you are buying the same foods you've bought before, and have already confirmed that the food is a good choice for you.

Better yet: buy whole foods whenever you can. If you avoid packaged foods, you won't need to spend your time reading labels.

BONUS HABIT #2
KEEP A FOOD DIARY

Few tips or practices are as universally applauded for losing weight as keeping a food diary. Writing down everything you eat and drink has many benefits including being realistic about what has gone into your mouth.

I have found that keeping a food diary is also very useful for sustainable weight control, especially during times when temptation seems to be all around. I don't always keep a food diary, but it is a practice that I start anytime my resolve to resist empty calories is slipping.

You will find this helpful, too. Especially if you really lean in and honestly write down everything you've eaten or had to drink, even that little mouthful of cookie that jumped into your mouth. Like me, you will find that writing everything down is a deterrent to eating unconsciously.

My careless eating and drinking habits clean up when a food diary notebook is in my purse.

There's ample scientific evidence that shows keeping a food diary works for weight loss

The Kaiser Center for Health Research conducted a six month study* of 1,700 people. Half of the study's participants, 850 people, kept a food diary and <u>lost twice as much weight</u> as the other half who did nothing to document their eating and drinking. *

Twice as much!

What other little technique will help you lose twice as much weight for your efforts?

I can't think of any. Keeping a food diary is a gentle daily practice. Yes, it takes discipline, but the benefits are very clear.

Don't buck the scientific findings. If you want to maximize your efforts at weight loss, and then later at weight control, become familiar with keeping a food diary.

*Weight loss during the intensive intervention phase of the weight-loss maintenance trial, by JF Hollis, Victor J. Stevens, PhD, senior investigator, Weight Loss Maintenance Trial Research Group, Kaiser Permanente Center for Health Research, Portland, Ore. Published August, 2008, American Journal of Preventive Medicine.

Food diaries help with portion control and mindless grazing

A food diary not only gives you a realistic overview of what you're actually eating, but it will also point out how much. Like many of you, I personally struggle with portion control, especially for foods I love. The act of actually documenting how much I'm eating can be shocking, actually, especially if I take the extra step of writing down the calories, as well as the quantity.

I tend to graze during the day, especially if I'm home and have unlimited access to my kitchen. Any walk through results in a quick nibble. My favorite nibble to grab is from a bag of jumbo raisins, or, sometimes I leave apple slices on the kitchen counter. These sound harmless, but a whole day of grazing damages my appetite for mealtimes. More importantly, continual grazing undermines my efforts at self-control.

Forcing myself to keep a food diary stops mindless grazing cold.

One important effect of keeping a food diary is that it will train you to think about what you're going to eat. That's right. It's not just about writing down what has already happened. If you accept and really do write down everything you eat, you will soon get in the habit of thinking "Do I really want that if I have to write it down?" It's really a wonderful tool to reinforce your self-control.

HERE ARE THE TOP REASONS TO KEEP A FOOD DIARY

If you need more persuasion than the truth that you can lose twice as much weight by keeping a food diary, here are some additional reasons.

REASON #1: Manage mindless eating

Are you sitting on the couch eating pretzels and chips while watching the game?

How about munching through that breadbasket at the restaurant? If you are really faithful about writing down every mouthful, you'll start to wonder why you're eating without really being aware of what you're doing. Control starts with awareness. Keeping a food diary will really help you identify what you're truly eating so you can do something positive about it.

REASON #2: Increase awareness of your nutrition

Are you really getting enough helpings of vegetables? Are you eating the fiber-rich foods you've promised yourself ? How about avoiding added sugars? Writing down what you've eaten then reviewing it will give you an accurate picture of how you are managing your nutritional needs.

You can include the water you are drinking and—very important—how much you have exercised every day.

If you want to increase the details, you can note carbohydrate and protein grams in addition to the usual calories and portion size notes.

REASON #3: Track your progress for inspiration and encouragement

When you're in the day-to-day routine of life, sometimes it's hard to feel that you've really been making progress. It can be very inspirational having a food diary available to show what you were doing a month ago vs what you are doing now.

Progress comes in small steps, usually, when it comes to changing your habits. We all want the giant, world-shaking transformation to make our futures better. But....sorry to be so realistic…there is no fairy godmother with a magic wand to wave over our bodies and our appetites. You must do it yourself, and a food diary is a marvelous way to track your progress. If you were to keep one for six months, then compare your last week with your first week, I bet that would feel like you have achieved a magic change.

REASON #4: You have the option of tracking your emotions while eating

If you're an emotional eater, this could be a huge breakthrough for you. If you are willing to consider then write down how you were feeling when you eat, this could give you some real insight.

Since this book contains a lot of my personal information, I don't mind sharing that I eat when I'm anxious. There is something about the mouth action that gives me comfort. For years I ate crackers and pretzels, mostly refined white flour. Now I eat sunflower seeds, one at a time. And I chew sugarless gum which has two benefits: I get the mouth action I need, and the gum's presence acts as a deterrent to putting anything else in my mouth.

REASON #5: You are holding yourself accountable

If you make a promise to yourself, does it matter less than a promise to someone else? No! What could be more important than a promise to yourself about your health? If you intend to lose weight, accountability is a primary tool. That's why programs like Weight Watchers have you weigh in every week.

There is power in being witnessed, even when the witness is yourself.

REASON #6: And don't forget: You'll lose twice as much weight!

Why make the effort to lose weight and not try to maximize your loss? The time spent will be the same. Avoid disappointment and get on board with keeping a food diary any time you are trying to take off some extra pounds.

HERE'S WHAT YOU SHOULD LOOK FOR IN A FOOD DIARY

Keeping a food diary doesn't need to be fancy. You could write everything down in a school notebook. Or, you could buy one of several styles of food diaries available on Amazon. If you're part of a program like Weight

Watchers, you already know that they have food diaries available and that using it is a big part of their program. That's because it works!

There are also food diary apps for your smart phone. If you don't want to mess around with paper, download one. I recommend the *Calorie Counter & Diet Tracker* by MyFitnessPal.com. And, it's free!

If you buy an existing food diary, take a look at how the pages are set up. Here is what you should see:

- Plenty of room to write down everything you eat, morning, afternoon and evening.

- Columns for entering quantity and calories eaten.

- A place to enter totals for calories.

- A place to enter the date and your weight at the start of the week.

- A place to enter exercise.

- A space to enter hours of sleep from the night before.

- Space to make comments about what you can do to improve.

- Space to write praise for your achievements.

- Boxes to check off for water, vegetable and fruit helpings.

It's helpful to also have a summary page for the week so you can see your progress.

Not many food diaries currently available on the market have a place to enter what you're feeling when you eat, or why you ate that item. I know that this is a sensitive area, but our emotions can make a huge difference in when and how much we are eating. If we can identify that we are using food for comfort, but that use is sabotaging our weight loss and control efforts, it's your signal to look for other ways to successfully comfort yourself. I struggle with emotional eating myself, so I've been there. And it's really true that you can expand your techniques for comfort and calm beyond eating. This is clearly the topic for a whole other book!

And, finally, a food diary will help you track if you are craving sugar

Keeping a list of everything you've eaten during the day is a clear road map on whether you have been able to move away from foods with added sugar. If you see that this is not happening, please go back and read *Habit #6: Avoid Added Sugars and Sweetened Drinks*, and also *Habit #10: Control Your Food Cravings*.

BONUS HABIT #3
REPEAT SUCCESSFUL MEALS

Repeating meals saves you time and money
Recipes for breakfast and lunch

When I first started writing this book, and showed the chapter titles to friends, many of them went right for the title of this Bonus Habit. Apparently repeating successful meals is highly desirable, but I got the idea that my friends were slightly embarrassed to be doing this. Could there be something about eating the same lunch, day after day, that people feel uncomfortable admitting?

We are always urged to try something new. Over 20,000 new packaged foods are introduced every year, and their producers want them to sell! Magazines push new recipes. There always seems to be a new, exciting flavor. Some new magic food that will improve our health.

It's great to be an adventurous eater and try new things. Just remember to use your common sense about any wild claims. But, if you're busy and trying to control your weight, just repeating a nutritious meal is a good way to go.

Repeating meals has many benefits:

- You will have planned ahead which helps control impulsive eating.

- You can anticipate that you'll enjoy the meal. Whether you'll like it or not won't be a mystery. You can trust your decisions.

- You already have experience with portion control.

- If you are counting calories, you have already done this and can just relax and eat.

- If you are buying food to prepare the meal, you know exactly what to get. This helps shorten your shopping time and also helps you anticipate your spending budget.

- If you are preparing the meal, you can make a larger quantity to be divided over several meals. This really helps save time and money.

- If you are buying the meal at a restaurant, deli or fast food outlet, you also know exactly what to expect. Hopefully, you're making a wise choice and avoiding added sugar and fat, and you are eating a high-fiber meal. (Adding a salad is a quick solution.)

I think that the primary benefit to repeating meals is that it helps you plan ahead. You've seen in this book that weight control benefits from planning ahead because impulsive decisions about food frequently damage your efforts. Knowing what you are going to eat helps you stay on track with your longterm goals.

Cooking large quantities in advance

Whenever possible, I will make either a large bowl of salad to keep in the refrigerator, a large casserole or a large vegetable stir fry on the stove top. Slow cookers are also a very useful tool for preparing food in advance. I like to have prepared food ready to scoop onto a plate then heated as necessary in the microwave. That way, I don't need to cook every day when I'm home. Some people enjoy preparing meals from scratch every day, but, regretfully, that's not me.

In the days when I left early for work, I could scoop my lunch into plastic carrying boxes. Coming home for dinner with prepared food ready and waiting for me made sitting down with my family easy. We all participated in cooking for the family on Sunday nights, making super large quantities so we could enjoy left over meals during the week. It wasn't hard to add a fresh side dish which added variety to our evening dinners.

Whether you live alone or with others, consider making extra quantities whenever you cook.

There are cookbook authors who have jumped on this trend. Just look for "Cooking For The Week" in your bookstore's cooking section. (Also see *Part Five: Resources*.) You can always increase the recipes for your favorite meals for multiple days of leftovers.

Breakfast is the perfect meal to repeat

Since breakfast is often the most rushed meal of the day, knowing in advance what you're going to eat is very helpful. If possible, make sure that your kitchen is stocked for at least a full week. I chose breakfast foods with a longer shelf life, so I don't have to worry about food staying fresh.

RECIPES:
TWO FAVORITE BREAKFASTS TO REPEAT

All recipes make one portion and are easy to increase by doubling or tripling ingredients

For most days when I'm home, I eat one of the two following breakfasts. Both offer protein, whole grain fiber, taste great and are fast to prepare. I've been eating these breakfasts for years and never get tired of them. As noted, you can easily add new ingredients to both for variety.

Shopping list for everything you need for the week and longer:

Here's a shopping list that will help you get ready to repeat the two breakfasts described below. These supplies will last you about two weeks:

For Egg Breakfasts:

- Eggs: 1 dozen

- Butter or butter substitute

- Whole grain rice cakes

- Lettuce: your favorite type

Optional:

- Fresh spinach: 1 lb

- Fresh mushrooms

- Fresh tomatoes

For Cereal Breakfasts :

- Whole grain hot cereal (or oatmeal): 1 lb container

- Pumpkin pie spice

- Apples: your favorite type

Optional:

- Almonds: slices or slivered,

- Plain Greek yogurt

EGG BREAKFAST:
Eggs with vegetables, scrambled or in a quick omelet

I vary how eggs are prepared but I always cook the yokes. (Just my preference.) To add vegetables to your eggs, cook them in the pan first until wilted, then break the eggs on top. Scramble right through the vegetables. While the pan is cooking, put a handful of lettuce and one rice cake or whole grain crackers on your plate. I pile the egg dish on top of the lettuce, for a beautiful, colorful pile of food.

As you will see, this is a very casual recipe, designed to produce a quick, nutritious breakfast with minimum fuss.

Tools needed:

- Non-stick frying pan

- Spatula to stir

- Teaspoon to measure butter/butter substitute/oil

- Knife if vegetables need cutting

- Plate

Ingredients:

- Two fresh eggs

- 1 tsp butter/butter substitute or vegetable oil

- 1 cup fresh vegetables of your choice (ex: spinach,

- mushrooms, tomatoes, zucchini)

- 1 cup lettuce to dress your plate

- Salt and pepper to taste

Step #1: Decide whether your eggs will be alone or with vegetables. Scrambled eggs without vegetables takes about four minutes.

To sauté the fresh vegetables first will add another four to six minutes.

Step #2: Put one scant teaspoon of butter, butter substitute or oil in your pan. Turn heat on high. When the oil is hot, add a handful of fresh mushrooms. After two minutes, stir the mushrooms and add a handful of spinach. Stir them together. The spinach will start to wilt immediately.

For variety, you can add any fresh vegetables. And, I often use dinner leftovers in my eggs! Just put a scoop in the pan, and heat them up.

Step #3: When what's the in the pan is hot, you can add the eggs. Either scramble them in a separate bowl then pour into the pan, or crack the eggs directly into the vegetable mix and scramble them in the pan.

Cook and stir over medium heat until eggs are firm.

Step #4: Prepare your breakfast plate with a handful of salad and a portion of whole grains. I prefer whole grain rice cakes, but whole grain toast or crackers are also fine.

Step #5: Arrange your egg dish on your plate, sit and enjoy your breakfast!

If you prefer the more elegant appearance of an omelet, follow all directions above to heat the vegetables, but remove them from the pan to a separate plate. Wipe the pan clean, and add just the barest amount of butter/butter substitute/oil. Heat the pan on high heat. Scramble your eggs in a separate bowl and pour into the pan as soon as it's hot. Rotate the pan and distribute the raw eggs to the sides, while lifting the part already cooked. This will help the eggs cook faster. When most of the eggs are cooked, turn the heat to medium and place your vegetables on JUST ONE SIDE of the eggs. That way, you can fold over the other side, making a tidy half-moon shaped omelet.

Arrange your attractive omelet on your plate with salad and whole grains and enjoy! Feel free to substitute apple or orange slices for the whole grains. Either way, you will be getting fiber and protein on your plate.

CEREAL BREAKFAST:
Whole grain cereal with fruit and yogurt

This is my favorite breakfast in cold weather, and it is surprisingly filling. This breakfast will last me three or four hours before hunger crosses my mind. The secret is choosing your whole grain cereal very carefully. Here's my absolute favorite:

- Trader Joe's Organic Multigrain Hot Cereal: 100% whole grain, rye, barley, oats & wheat.

Not only is it delicious, but it's very inexpensive, about $3.00 per container (1 lb 2 oz.) It keeps for weeks. It only takes 1/3 cup to make a hearty breakfast for one person, and my recipe will easily scale up to prepare breakfast for more people.

NOTE: This cereal does not keep well once it's cooked. Prepare only what you need for each meal.

Tools needed:

- Medium sized, microwave safe soup bowl

- Measuring cup or scoop that shows 1/3 cup

- Microwave, but you could cook this on your stove top.

Ingredients:

- 1/3 cup whole grain cereal, dry and ready to cook

- Apple: ½ if large, 1 whole if small

- ½ tsp Pumpkin pie spice

- ½ cup Water

- Optional:

- 1/3 cup plain Greek yogurt

- 1 tbsp Almonds, sliced or slivered

To prepare in the microwave:

Step #1: Choose a bowl with sides at least 4 inches high. You could prepare the hot cereal directly in the bowl you'll be eating from, or a serving bowl. Just make sure that the bowl is deep enough to hold the cereal, the chopped apple and the water which will boil.

Step #2: Chop your apple. I like small pieces because they will cook faster. Usually, I leave the skin on. (And remove the core, of course.)

Put the apple pieces in the bowl and sprinkle with the pumpkin pie spice. You'll be surprised that this makes the cereal taste like apple pie. What a treat for breakfast!

Step #3: Measure 1/3 cup of dried cereal and place it in the bowl. Do not stir yet.

Step #4: Measure ½ cup of water and pour it over the cereal, apples and spice. Now, stir. The water should be ½ inch above the dry ingredients. If it's not, add more. If you prefer your hot cereal somewhat soupy, add more water as desired.

Step #5: Microwave on high for 5 minutes. Let cool for 2 minutes when finished. (I use this time to get dressed and ready.)

Beware of using a bowl that is too shallow. Cleaning your microwave after the cereal boils over is a hassle. When in doubt, chose a larger bowl.

Step #6: Add yogurt to the top of your cereal. Sprinkle with almonds as desired. Sometimes I add soymilk, too.

If you have a jar of fruit-only preserves, add a teaspoon for variety. Occasionally adding a teaspoon of honey is acceptable. Never add sugar. Try to adapt your taste to the apples and spices which have a natural sweetness.

Sit down with your bowl of goodness and enjoy! When I was super rushed in the morning, I made this cereal in a plastic bowl (very helpful since it didn't get hot in the microwave) then took it with me in the car to eat while I commuted by car. Not the most enjoyable way to have breakfast, but it was very efficient. I was fed, satisfied and ready to face my workday.

To prepare on the stove top:

Assemble all ingredients in the order listed above in a medium sized pot. Heat on high until water starts to boil, then turn down to simmer. Simmer for 5 minutes. Serve as described above.

WHAT ABOUT LUNCH?
All recipes make one portion and are easy to increase by doubling or tripling ingredients

I think that lunch is possibly the most dangerous meal for weight control because it's the time of day that you are most likely to be out of your home and facing temptations. It's important that you make every effort to control what you are eating mid-day, regardless of whether you bring your lunch or go find it. This is especially true if you are in a weight losing stage. As always, the more fiber in your food, the more full you will feel and the more stable your blood sugar will be for the longest time.

It's not always practical to have enough time in the morning to dress, get the family ready, make breakfast then also make yourself a lunch to take. If you're working away from home, chances are that you eat your workday lunches out. You could be lucky enough to live walking distance to home, but most of us need to deal with finding a meal in the middle of the day.

My husband works at a large, multi-national company with a campus removed from any shopping districts. The company provides a very well-stocked cafeteria with many healthy choices. He takes a mid-morning and mid-afternoon snack from home, but always eats his lunch at the cafeteria.

When I was working, my company was much smaller and did not provide lunches, although there was a lunchroom with a refrigerator, microwaves and a hot plate. Over the years when I was figuring out which habits would be most successful for weight control, I experimented with many different lunches, from frozen meals to boxes of dinner leftovers. But, it wasn't until I stumbled upon two different styles of lunches that I could easily repeat that my lunch habits fell into place.

Generally, I believe that your weight control efforts will be more successful, especially while you are learning new habits, if you control your lunches by bringing them from home.

Here are my two favorite lunches to take to repeat.

272

WRAP LUNCH:
Fill a whole grain wrap for a delicious sandwich

Wraps are an especially useful way to taking leftovers to work. They eliminate the need for containers and utensils, and are incredibly flexible about which ingredients to include. You can add strong flavors with just a little bit of condiment spread on the wrap, and pile on the fiber by adding lettuce or vegetables.

The all-popular burrito is a wrap, but—in case you didn't know—the beans most often used in burritos are very high in fat, possibly from lard. You know by now to be vigilant about hidden fats and sugar. Making your own wraps is the best way to get a "the most nutrition bang for your calorie buck".

Flat breads that are pliable are a better weight control choice for sandwiches than slices of bread, because they have fewer calories and carbohydrates. These days, there are many choices of tortillas available at most food retailers. Try to find one that is made from organic ingredients and is whole grain. My favorite is the organic tortilla made with olive oil.

Tools needed:

- Cutting board or work surface
- Knife for spreading soft ingredients
- Sharp knife for cutting hard ingredients
- Plastic wrap to make transport easy
- or: plate for immediate serving.

Ingredients:

- 1 whole grain wrapper
- 1 tsp of condiment such as mustard, wasabi, non-fat mayonnaise, pesto, curry sauce
- 3 oz sliced meat, egg, tuna fish, tofu or other protein
- ½ cup of vegetable or salad

Step #1: Lay out the wrapper nice and flat. Make sure there is no moisture underneath it, otherwise it will get soggy and hard to remove from the work surface.

Step #2: Spread your condiments equally all over the wrapper.

Step #3: Slice your protein and lay it out evenly in the middle of the wrapper, in a straight line about 3" across. If the round wrapper were a clock, imagine that you are spreading protein between 9:00 and 3:00 o'clock. Leave about 1" at either end to help you fold the wrapper without the ingredients falling out.

Step #4: Lay on the vegetables or salad evenly in the middle of the wrapper, on top of your protein.

Step #5: Fold and roll the wrapper the long way, starting with 6:00, then 12:00. Tuck in other ends. Press them firmly to make sure they hold.

SALAD LUNCH:
Arrange your toppings for a beautiful presentation and wonderful flavors

My family calls this "Refrigerator Cleanout Salad" because I typically put salad greens on a plate then pile on whatever leftovers happen to be in the refrigerator. I am careful about portion control, but I do like many different flavors on top of my greens. Sometimes it's leftover rotisserie chicken with a scoop of brown rice or quinoa. I always chop salad vegetables like cucumbers, celery and tomatoes to add, and then sprinkle the top with almonds, sunflower seeds or a small portion of feta cheese.

The secret is to keep your salad dressing very controlled. Try putting it in a small, separate bowl and dipping your fork in with every other bite.

Sometimes I run a contest with myself to see if I can create a "Seven Ingredient Salad": including no less than seven toppings.

Here are some possible toppings:

- Leftover dinner meat (3 oz)
- Sliced chicken, beef, pork, tofu, tempeh, fish (3 oz)

- Boiled egg
- Chopped apple
- Sliced cucumber
- Cherry tomatoes
- Sliced grapes
- Sliced celery
- Sliced carrots
- Sliced red, green or yellow peppers
- Fresh peas (green, snow, snap)
- Corn kernels
- Onions (yellow, red, green)
- Sliced fennel
- Leftover whole grains (1/4 cup)
- Potato salad (2 oz)
- Egg salad (2 oz)
- Sliced nuts
- Seeds (sunflower, pumpkin)
- Crumbled cheese (1 oz)
- Cottage cheese (2 oz)
- Sliced pickles
- Capers

I love making these composed salads for how beautiful fresh vegetable colors can be arranged on the plate. There's nothing like a bed of greens to show off toppings at their best.

Explore different types of greens

When I was growing up, the only lettuce my mother used was iceberg. I loved the crunch but it was definitely lacking in flavor. When romaine lettuce became popular, I cried for joy and feasted on Caesar salads.

Today, there is a much wider understanding that fresh greens are a very healthy choice and spring greens, kale and fresh spinach have become very popular.

Consider trying new types of greens and explore their flavors. Arugula and radicchio top my list for slightly tart and peppery greens. Butter lettuce has a sweet taste. Tight lettuce heads like iceberg tend to be crisper, while loose leaf greens tend to have a wider variety of flavors, depending on the type.

Here are some different types of greens to look for. Please ask your grocer to widen the selection of greens in the store if you don't see them.

- Kale
- Spinach
- Butter lettuce (bibb or Boston)
- Spring mix (sold in package)
- Arugula (also known as rocket)
- Radicchio
- Escarole
- Cress
- Oak leaf
- Romaine
- Endive
- Baby beet greens
- Frisée (also known as chicory)
- Gem

Tools needed:
- Cutting board or work surface
- Medium sized bowl or large plate
- Sharp knife
- Optional: Grater to grate cheese

Ingredients:

- 1 to 2 cups of salad greens. More is better.

- 2 to 3 oz of protein (meat, fish, tofu, etc.)

- ¼ cup each of 3 to 4 vegetables, cooked or raw

- 2 tbsp each of nuts or seeds

- 1 to 2 tbsp salad dressing

- Optional: 1 oz grated cheese

- ¼ cup of 1 fruit

Step #1: Place greens on your plate. No need to measure. More is better. Cover the entire plate with greens. You should have nice mound that rises in the middle.

Step #2: Assuming your plate is round, Lay your protein at 12:00 high.

Step #3: Arrange your other ingredients, going around the plate like hands on a clock. Take a moment to look at your composition and admire the colors and textures.

Step #4: Sprinkle topping like nuts, seeds, grated cheese, capers over the mound of your salad.

Step #5: Consider your salad dressing carefully. Don't ruin your work at portion control by drowning your salad with flavored oil. A light sprinkle of plain olive oil and vinegar is all you really need. If you use a pre-mixed dressing, read the label to look for hidden sugars.

Salads can be works of art, but sometimes our taste needs training

Not all of us naturally love green salads. Some of us prefer salads that are heavy on mayonaise like potato salad and egg salad. If that's your preference, consider trying to train yourself to eat these over a bed of greens. You will get more fiber, feel more full longer, and over time, cut calories as you increase the amount of greens while decrease the amount of high-calorie mayonaise-y salads.

My husband is very fussy about the greens he eats, and has an aversion to greens that are bitter. He refuses to eat many of the wonderful mixes of arugula, radicchio and frisée greens that I love, so for our meals together, I stick to romaine and butter lettuces for him.

If you also find lettuce to be bitter, try these sweeter varieties:

- Romaine
- Gem
- Butter

A whole head of romaine lettuce only has 15 calories!

Do not give up on salad greens. For weight control, they are a practical way to stretch the volume that you're eating so you can eat more without gaining weight. There is no other food you can put in your mouth that will give you the same satisfying combination of crunch, chew, swallow, fiber, flavor and low, low calories.

One excellent weight control trick is to lay a bed of greens on your plate then place your main dishes on top. This makes the plate look very full and appealing, so if you're struggling to accept portion control, it's a way to create what looks like a huge portion for very few calories.

You can even grill some of the types with tighter heads! Grilled radicchio is a gourmet delight. I love grilled gem lettuce because it has a naturally sweet flavor and needs little sauce.

Salad greens are virtually a free food for weight control. Eat as much as you'd like, all day, every day.

BONUS HABIT #4
FORGIVE YOURSELF
& START AGAIN

**You deserve praise for working to improve your health
If you stumble, just recommit to your longterm goal
of weight control and move forward
Never give up!**

Eating is often an emotional act. We eat for comfort when we're lonely, upset or anxious. We eat to make ourselves feel better. Sometimes, we eat because everyone around us is eating and we want to be part of the group, even if we know that the food served won't be healthy for us.

And, there are times when we're so busy that we just grab what's convenient. Thanks to packaged foods and fast food outlets, this has become so easy to do. It seems like there's a candy bar, soda or hamburger just around the corner wherever we are. So many convenient foods are packed with added sugar, salt and fat, that it's easy to sabotage our best intentions.

So…our short-term actions are sometimes in conflict with our longterm goals.

Weight control is a longterm goal. It's not a ten day cleansing diet where if you "cheat" for two days, you've blown 20% of your effort. There is no "cheating" in the lifestyle of weight control. There are mistakes, definitely, but understanding that the transition to a new lifestyle takes practice and time, grant yourself a built-in attitude of forgiveness as you are learning.

You deserve forgiveness when you are trying to master something new.

Forgiveness but not forgetfulness. We all make mistakes. If you are serious about weight control, you do not forget your goal is to learn a new lifestyle that will take off your extra weight and keep it off while making you more aware of your food environment. You will be developing the tools to be able to protect and control yourself from behaviors that are unhealthy and do not promote weight control.

That this will require repeated practice cannot be overstated. To learn something new, you must do it over and over. If you've ever studied music, you know this. If you've ever been involved with sports, you know this. Learning weight control habits is no different.

It takes me between 15 and 20 times, practicing the same thing to finally get comfortable and do it almost automatically. In a practical world, it might look like this:

You walk into the office lunchroom. There's a tray of donuts. You love glazed donuts, but you look away and don't take one. It's hard. You really want it but you're strong. The next day, the same thing happens, and it's also hard to walk away. All week long, you are painfully resisting that glazed donut. Then, the next week, it seems less painful. It's easier to turn away. The following week, you see the tray but somehow that burning desire has faded. And, finally, in week four, you can walk into a room with donuts and it's just a room. You go straight to the coffee and shrug at the donuts. They don't call to you. The pain is gone. The desire is gone.

What's happened is that you have reinforced the habit of refusing donuts. You have built a new brain pathway that says "I will skip the donut" which substitutes for the brain pathway which says "Take the donut". You have practiced at least fifteen times and now you can refuse the donut with ease. You have mastered being strong and choosing to protect your longterm health over a couple of minutes of taste pleasure.

Does three weeks of practice seem like it's insurmountably long? Don't forget that you are building habits for THE REST OF YOUR LIFE. Three weeks is, hopefully, just a blip of time compared to your longterm future.

Always keep a perspective about time.

Don't beat yourself up for mistakes.
Just get on with the good habits.

There is no failure as long as your commitment to your longterm health remains strong. There are only slip-ups. Most of us have been on diet programs, then fallen off and feel just hopeless about it. It's a horrible feeling, mixing guilt and shame and just wanting to give up. Grabbing for comfort food to make ourselves feel better, after failing miserably at staying on a diet, is an understandable reaction.

I know the feeling well, having fallen off numerous diets in my 35 years of yo-yo craziness. Even though I was able to stick with some programs for weeks, and even achieve my goal weight for a while, there were others that I started on Monday and had fallen off by Wednesday.

But, here's the difference between a diet and a weight control lifestyle: you are choosing to reinvent your life <u>permanently</u>—not signing up for a temporary program. You understand that it will take time to internalize new habits and that practice is necessary. If you overeat high-calorie food on Monday, you know that you must return to portion control and better choices on Tuesday.

You might take a detour, but you haven't ended the journey.

You have the guide for where you need to go in the 10 Daily Habits. You can always return to it. The 10 Daily Habits are your foundation. It doesn't go away with one or two missteps.

Never give up.

First, what is a mistake? Let's call it a "stumble",
so you understand that it's just a misstep
and you can keep on going.

When you're creating a new lifestyle, the days are long and the weeks and months stretch ahead. There are temptations, and times when you fall off the program. It happens. Do your best to get back on track as soon as you can. We all stumble occasionally, even frequently. But if you are moving in the general direction of absorbing the 10 Daily Habits, a few stumbles here and there won't kill your longterm progress.

Believe in the longterm and don't give up.

Here's the list of the top ten stumbles that work against a weight control lifestyle:

These are, of course, just the flipside of the 10 Daily Habits. In the individual chapters about every habit, there are details about why each habit is important for weight loss and control, and what you can do to learn and maintain it. There's a tremendous amount of information in this book to remember and to put into action. It's understandable to make slips and stumbles over the weeks that you are learning. And, even months later, when you are comfortable living with the 10 Daily Habits, it's certainly possible to slip up. Nobody's perfect but you can always keep trying.

Stumble #1: Not getting enough sleep.

You'll have less willpower and self control because your brain won't be rested.

See *Habit #1: Get Enough Sleep* for more information.

Stumble #2: Not eating breakfast

By not jump-starting your metabolism in the morning, you risk crashing and eating foolishly later in the day.

See *Habit #2: Start the Day Well with a Breakfast of Protein and Whole Grains* for more information.

Stumble #3: Not exercising for more than two days.

Without movement, your metabolism slows down, and your muscles lose their strength and mass. Because muscles are the most metabolically active tissue in your body and will use more calories than any other body part, it's important to keep your muscles toned and strong.

Even if you can't schedule 30 minutes for exercise, you can always fidget or wiggle or march in place to keep your body moving. Don't give up exercise for more than two days in a row! It's essential that you are not sedentary. Do whatever you need to do to inspire yourself. An exercise buddy or walking partner, a pedometer to measure steps with a goal of 10,000 steps every day are both useful to keep you moving.

Staying active is critical for weight control.

See *Habit #3: Exercise for 30 Minutes Every Day* for more information.

Stumble #4: Forgetting to be vigilant about portion control.

If you binge or gorge on a high-calorie food, resolve to do better next time. It happens. Do your best to make these isolated events.

Consider not putting yourself in the position to be offered such a large volume of temptation.

Don't sabotage yourself with repeated episodes of binging, and if you do, think about getting help for this kind of behavior. Remember that each time you resist, you build the habit of saying "no". The more times you say "no", the easier it gets because, internally, you are actually saying "yes" I can take care of my health. "Yes" I am strong. "Yes" I can trust myself. Build your trust in yourself, one decision at a time.

See *Habit #4: Learn and Practice Portion Control* and *Habit #10: Control Your Food Cravings* for more information.

Stumble #5: Eating something from a package without reading the label.

Not being aware of what you're putting in your body is dangerous for weight control. Do your best to learn about what makes up the food you eat and don't put anything in your mouth without being aware of what it is. Of course the easiest way to not read food labels is to stay away from packaged products and eat whole foods!

See *Habit #5: Know what's in Your Food Before You Put It in Your Mouth* for more information.

Stumble #6: Eating sugary foods or drinking sweetened drinks or sodas.

Eating sugar is a huge subject with many implications for your health. For many reasons, it's very hard to avoid eating sugar and even worse, wanting to eat sugar, but it is possible. Switch to high-fiber foods, which take longer to digest, keeping you feeling full and satisfied longer.

See *Habit #6: Avoid Added Sugars and Sweetened Drinks* for more information.

Stumble #7: Eating refined white flour: pasta, white bread or pastries, cake.

Refined white flour is all around us, from pretzels to spaghetti to croissants. It's hard to avoid but at least it's not hidden.

If you have gone gluten-free, you have a head start because most refined white flour is made from wheat. For the rest of us who eat wheat, it's important to seek out whole grains. Note that "whole wheat" does not mean "whole grain". Only whole grain contains all the natural parts of the original grain and has not been tampered with by removing the bran and the germ. Whole grain baked goods are not always easy to find, but they're worth the effort for the extra vitamins, minerals and fiber. You just get more nutritional "bang" for your calorie "buck". Refined white flour is basically empty calories.

See *Habit #7: Find Substitutes for Refined White Flour* for more information.

Stumble #8: Going too long between meals or snacks.

Your brain requires glucose for energy, which comes from the food you eat and travels to your brain in your bloodstream. (This is your blood sugar level.) If you skip meals, you run the risk of having your blood sugar levels dip so low that you become desperate for food and won't be able to make wise decisions, or wait to find healthy food. This is especially dangerous for weight control when we're super hungry because sugary snacks and fast foods are so easily available.

The two solutions are to plan ahead to have healthy snacks ready and don't skip meals. Eat high-fiber, low sugar foods for your meals and snacks so you don't have a sugar crash. Remember, fiber only comes from plants. Pay attention to protein, from both plant and animal sources for breakfast, which is especially helpful to jumpstart your metabolism after you've been sleeping.

See *Habit #8: Snack Often* for more information.

Stumble #9: Forgetting to notice the pleasure and beauty around you.

Beating yourself up for errors and omissions is easy, and many of us who struggle with our weight are very self-critical. And yet there are pleasures available if we can just get away from our critical inner voices. Stop and take time to tune into what you touch, what you hear, what you smell and what you can see. Seek out beauty and pleasure as an antidote to criticism. Then praise yourself for having found it.

See *Habit #9: Enjoy at Least One Non-Caloric Pleasure Every Day* for more information.

Stumble #10: Binging on sugary or fatty foods.

We all have cravings. We must learn to be realistic and deal with them in order to control our weight for life. Does it matter if you binge on pizza one time? Not much. But what about day after day? You'll sabotage your efforts to lose weight and keep if off if you can't control your cravings. Basically, an occasional stumble, not a big deal. Stumbling and overeating frequently, you're in weight control trouble. It's time to look for help.

You can diminish your cravings with practice and by being prepared. (Ex: Remove tempting food from your home and do not buy it.) I also found tremendous help with hypnosis therapy to control cravings.

See *Habit #10: Control Your Food Cravings* for more information.

HOW REALISTIC IS IT TO ACTUALLY LIVE ALL 10 HABITS EVERY DAY?

Yes, it can be done but all days are opportunities for a variety of behaviors. Even the best intentions are not met sometimes. Our days contain surprises, which is why planning ahead is so important to support your weight control efforts. Preparing healthy food, scheduling time to exercise and avoiding sugar and refined white flour (both simple carbohydrates) all contribute to comfortably moving through whatever the day throws at you.

Here's a big tip: Print off copies of the 10 Daily Habits Weekly Worksheet and keep it where you will see it frequently. Check off any habit you have practiced at least once that day. As your check marks fill the sheet, you will be surprised by your progress. When you see that any habit is not being checked off, this is your red flag to review that chapter and double-down on your effort.

And…things happen. There's a lot to keep track of. If your intention is to practice all 10 Daily Habits, you can be very forgiving of yourself if you drop the ball on one or two.

Even I am not perfect in my daily life when it comes to practicing each and every daily habit every single day. But, I do follow the majority of habits every day. At least 50% of the time, I manage to follow all 10 Daily Habits all day long.

So, what happens when I "blow it"? I acknowledge it, take responsibility and resolve to do better tomorrow.

That's the secret: Understand what you did and resolve to do better tomorrow.

Try to minimize the actions which put you in conflict with the 10 Daily Habits. For example: if you have a large plate of regular pasta, and you want to do it again, have a smaller plate, then a smaller one after that. Portion control is always the answer when you feel you must eat simple carbohydrates. (Or, better yet, find whole grain pasta.)

One bite of chocolate won't rock your world, but eating that whole box of chocolates will.

Are you sabotaged by food manufacturers that aggressively market sugary, fatty and salty foods?

Food manufacturers need to sell their products, and doing whatever they can to persuade you to buy and eat them is essential for corporate profits. May I suggest that you would be well advised to learn more about how the American food supply is formulated to grab your attention and enhance your desire? (You will find recommended books about this in *Part Five: Resources for Learning More*.)

The human brain reacts to sugar like it reacts to a drug. Excess sugar in your bloodstream travels to the brain where it's the trigger to release excess levels of dopamine, the powerful neurotransmitter that creates feelings of pleasure. The problem with continued consumption of sugar is that the brain starts to depend on it in order to maintain dopamine levels. Then, when sugar isn't present in your bloodstream, as dopamine levels fall, you feel moody, irritable, edgy and frustrated. This is the classic "sugar crash".

Remember that it's only been recently in human history that sugar has been widely distributed. For millions of years, we evolved without eating any added sugar whatsoever because it didn't exist. Sugar wasn't cultivated on a wide scale until the 1600's, and the invention of high fructose corn syrup wasn't until the 1970's. We can get along very well without any added sugar at all.

Sadly, in the 21st century, products with added sugar positively surround us, and if you are accustomed to eating or drinking them, stopping is not easy. Your brain has grown accustomed to reacting to frequent consumption of sugar and the release of dopamine feels good. It has been suggested that constant consumption of sugar creates an addiction-like condition, making withdrawal especially difficult.

If your daily diet includes packaged or fast foods with a lot of sugar, be aware that changing over to a diet of whole foods is not just a matter of developing different tastes. There is a physiological response that is experienced when someone transitions from a high sugar to a low sugar diet.

Forgive yourself for sugar cravings. Consider a sugar detox plan.

You can see now how sugar cravings aren't just imaginary. They are the result of actual chemical reactions in your brain. But, the good news is this: How to transition out of a high sugar diet is a very popular subject these days. There is a wealth of available information, usually under the title "Sugar detox".

A full sugar detox plan is not within the scope of this book, but these are easy to find. Just Google "sugar detox".

I've also included books about sugar detox in the *Resources* section.

You should ask your doctor if starting on this is a good idea for you. He/she may have one to recommend.

What's important here is that you can be realistic and start forgiving yourself for losing control and binging on sweetened foods. But being realistic also means that you must take action to improve your life and move away from excessive amounts of this powerful substance: sugar.

What alters your judgment? Alcohol?

Drinking alcohol is well known to alter your judgment and self-control. Plus, those drinks are basically empty calories, simple carbohydrates that also raise your blood sugar level. Like any other substance with empty calories, limiting your portions is absolutely essential for a weight control lifestyle.

Does drinking affect how much you eat? When you have wine, beer or spirits, do you go back for second portions or eat that extra dessert? Notice whether you are binging more, exercising less or not paying attention to portion control after you've been drinking.

If your drinking is excessive, that is a problem beyond the scope of this book. Please consider getting help.

What about strong emotions and eating? Do you binge when you're upset?

I heard terrible health news about one of my young children some years ago. That afternoon is now a horrible blur in my memory. During the course of his problem, which lasted three months, I gained 30 pounds, comforting myself with mountains of food. It was a 90 day eating binge during which I seemed to have no self-control. These were the days before I had formulated the 10 Daily Habits, and I was completely without any weight control foundation for a healthy lifestyle. I was lost in the wilderness of fear and worry about my child. Thank goodness he recovered completely.

Since then, over the almost twenty years that I have been living the 10 Daily Habits, there have been stressful times. My house burned down in a California wildfire. Both of my parents died. My longtime husband and I divorced. I had my own health issue. But the foundation provided by the 10 Daily Habits kept me on track. I still eat for comfort, but it's no longer out of control, and I choose foods that are healthier.

Following the 10 Daily Habits and believing in them over the years has really paid off.

Never give up! Write a weight control mission statement to keep yourself motivated.

It's a perilous world out there for weight control. Parties with cake, candy bars on every corner, restaurants selling you desserts, sodas, fast food that's fried, co-workers with donuts and cheap pizzas. And glorious buffets. Sometimes it seems as though the food you should resist far outnumbers the healthy food you should be eating.

No one is immune from temptation. What's a carrot compared to a piece of carrot cake?

I've stumbled off the 10 Daily Habits plenty of times. The holiday meal, the vacation, the wedding banquet. There are so many opportunities to indulge in rich, pleasurable foods.

But, I haven't waivered on what I've truly wanted longterm, and I remember it by saying this mission statement to myself whenever I feel my resolve slipping.

I will do my best to support my good health by taking good care of my body with healthy food, exercise, enough sleep and a realistic understanding of the challenges I face. I know I can master the habits I need to maintain a healthy weight for the rest of my life.

Consider writing a weight control mission statement for yourself:

____

____

____

____

____

The best mission statements are short and to the point. Mine is 52 words, and it took some time to organize my thoughts into a clear statement. You are welcome to borrow it for your own. If you do want to write one, expect that it will take some focus. It's a terrific opportunity to clearly declare your goals, and you may surprise yourself if you're absolutely truthful. I was surprised because it was finally time for me to let go of worrying about how thin I look as my top priority, and instead accept that protecting my metabolism and longterm health is so much more important.

I sincerely hope that offering you this book has had a positive influence on your commitment to your health and well-being.

Never take your eyes off the longterm goal.

NEVER. GIVE. UP.

PART FIVE:

RESOURCES
FOR LEARNING MORE

CURIOSITY IS YOUR BEST FRIEND

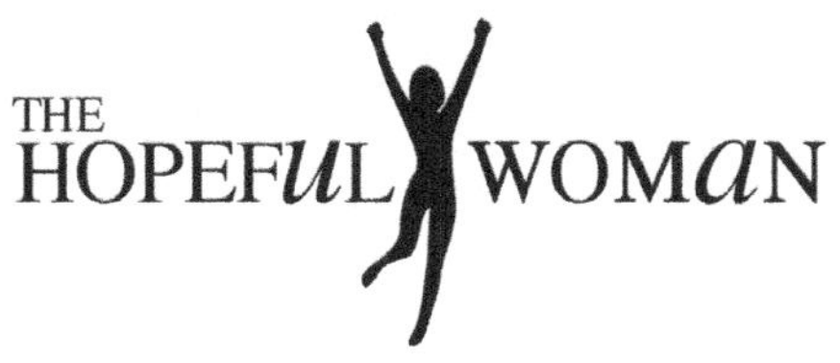

RECOMMENDED BOOKS

I recommend building a library of useful books that you can refer to when you have questions about nutrition, diet, metabolism and what to eat to stay healthy. I've sorted through hundreds of books to find ones from the most highly qualified and trustworthy authors. All are available on Amazon.

In addition, I've included carefully selected books about willpower, exercise, the American food system, and recommended books on the history of foods. The histories are very enjoyable to read, and you may be surprised at the complexities involved to develop the food and drinks we have available today.

Expand your knowledge with these good books.

Eating: The science of what to eat and what not to eat

These books focus on nutrition, how food is metabolized and how our bodies work. They are valuable reference books. You can often find immediate answers to your nutrition and dietary questions by checking with these highly qualified and trustworthy authors. I especially recommend the well-researched books by Marion Nestle and Gary Taubes, who are excellent writers.

- *What to Eat* by Marion Nestle

  North Point Press (a division of Farrar, Straus and Giroux) 2006

- *Why We Get Fat and What To Do About It* by Gary Taubes

  Anchor Books (a division of Random House, Inc.) 2010

- *Why Calories Count: From Science to Politics* by Marion Nestle and Malden Nesheim

  University of California Press 2012

- *Fat Chance: Beating the Odds Against Sugar, Processed Food, Obesity, and Disease* by Robert H. Lusting, M.D., M.S.L.

  Plume (Published by the Penguin Group) 2012

- *The End of Overeating: Taking Control of the Insatiable American Appetite* by David A. Kessler, M.D.

  Rodale 2009

- *Mindless Eating: Why We Eat More Than We Think* by Brian Wansink, PhD

  Bantam Books 2006

- *In Defense of Food: An Eater's Manifesto* by Michael Pollan

  The Penguin Press 2008

- *The Plant-Based Journey: A step-by-Step Guide for Transitioning to a Healthy Lifestyle and Achieving Your Ideal Weight* by Lani Muelrath

  BenBella Books, Inc. 2015

- *Gulp: Adventures on The Alimentary Canal* by Mary Roach

  W.W.Norton & Company 2013

Essential Food Counters

All of these books are small and easy to carry in your purse. Everyone trying to lose and control their weight should have a calorie counter as a handy reference.

- *Calorie, Fat & Carbohydrate Counter* by The Calorie King

  Family Health Publications 2012

- *The Glycemic Load Counter: A Pocket Guide to GL and GI Values for over 800 Foods* by Dr. Mabel Blades

  Ulysses Press 2008

- *DietMinder: Personal Food & Fitness Journal*

  A Deluxe Food Diary by F.E.Wilikins Diary 2001

The American Food System

These books are informative and will broaden your knowledge about the American food system. To be an informed consumer, it's important to understand the food supply chain and why foods are offered to you in markets and restaurants. You will learn a lot from reading any of these.

- *Fast Food Nation: The Dark Side of the All-American Meal* by Eric Schlosser

  Perennial (an imprint of Harper Collins Publishers) 2002

- *The Omnivore's Dilemma: A Natural History of Four Meals* by Michael Pollan

  The Penguin Press 2006

- *Food Politics: How The Food Industry Influences Nutrition and Health* by Marian Nestle

  University of California Press 2013 Revised edition

- *Salt Sugar Fat: How the Food Giants Hooked Us* by Michael Moss

  Random House 2014

Cookbooks: Cook for the whole week, and spiralizing vegetables

These books offer helpful techniques to make preparing nutritious meals easier. *Inspiralized* is an international best seller, describing innovative and delicious ways to cook vegetables.

- *Cook Once a Week* by Theresa Albert

  HaperCollins Publishers Ltd 2005

- *Cooking for The Week: Leisurely Weekend Cooking for Easy Weekday Meals* by Diane Morgan, Dan Taggart and Kathleen Taggart

  Chronicle Books 1999

- *Inspiralized: Turn Vegetables into Healthy, Creative, Satisfying Meals* by Ali Maffucci

  Clarkson Potter 2015

The history of agriculture, beverages and foods

These entertaining and informative books focus on the history of what we eat and drink, how we grow, trade and prepare our foods and beverages. Some of these histories will surprise you, especially the stories of beer, wine, coffee, tea, distilled spirits and Coca-Cola in *A History of the World in 6 Glasses*.

- *Sugar: A Bittersweet History* by Elizabeth Abbott

  Duckworth Overlook 2009

- *A History of The World in 6 Glasses* by Tom Standage

  Walker Publishing Company 2006

- *The True History of Chocolate* by Sophie D. Coe and Michael D. Coe

  Thames & Hudson 2013

- *Cooked: A Natural History of Transformation* by Michael Pollan

  Penguin Books 2014

- *Pure and Modern Milk: An Environmental History since 1900* by Kendra Smith-Howard

  Oxford University Press 2013

- *Meathooked: The History and Science of Our 2.5-Million-Year Obsession with Meat* by Marla Zaraska

  Basic Books 2016

Exercise

You probably have your favorite exercise DVDs or programs to watch. Or, perhaps you already go to a gym. If not, these are two useful books that can help you exercise at home. There are plenty of illustrations and photos to describe all moves.

- *Fit Quickies: 5-Minute Targeted Body-Shaping Workouts* by Lani Muelrath

  Alpha Books: Penguin Group 2013

- *Body for Life for Women: A Woman's Plan for Physical and Mental Transformation* by Pamela Peeke, M.D., M.P.H., F.A.C.P.

  Rodale Inc. 2005

Willpower and self-control

Everyone wants more willpower, and scientists are just starting to understand how it works. These books will help you understand, too.

- *Willpower: Rediscovery the Greatest Human Strength* by Roy F. Baumeister and John Tierney

  Penguin Books 2011

- *The Willpower Instinct: How Self-Control Works, Why It Matters, and What You Can Do to Get More of It* by Kelly McGonigal, PhD

  Avery (The Penguin Group) 2012

The obesity epidemic and diabetes

These books focus on how to actions we can take individually and collectively as a society to curb the rise of obesity and diabetes.

- *The End of Diabetes: The Eat to Live Plan to Prevent and Reverse Diabetes* by Joel Fuhrman

  HarperOne 2014

- *A Big Fat Crisis: The Hidden Forces Behind the Obesity Epidemic and How We Can End It* by Deborah A Cohen, M.D.

  Nation Books (Perseus Books Group) 2014

- *Diabesity: The Obesity-Diabetes Epidemic That Threatens America— And What We Must to Stop It* by Francine R. Kaufman, M.D.

  Bantam Dell 2005

FREE VIDEOS AVAILABLE ONLINE

Need a quick shot of motivation or an exercise program? Or, perhaps you'd like to go to a university-level lecture on health. These videos will educate and motivate you.

- *Sugar: The Bitter Truth* by Robert Lustig, M.D.

  University of California Television (UCTV)

  https://www.youtube.com/watch?v=dBnniua6-oM

- *The Skinny on Obesity* by Robert Lustig, M.D.

  University of California Television (UCTV)

  https://www.youtube.com/watch?v=moQZd1-BC0Y

- *Why We Get Fat: The Diet/Weight Relationship, An Alternative Hypothesis* by Gary Taubes

  The Science Media Production Center at Cornell

  https://www.youtube.com/watch?v=qEuIlQONcHw

- *Is a Calorie a Calorie? Processed Food, Experiment Gone Wrong* by Stanford Health Care

  https://www.youtube.com/watch?v=nxyxcTZccsE

- The Principles of a Healthy Diet: How Do We Know What to Eat? by Robert Baron, M.D.

  University of California Television (UCTV)

  https://www.youtube.com/watch?v=yN_BRYfpGAM

- *Why dieting doesn't usually work* – A TED Talk by Sandra Aamodt

  http://www.ted.com/talks/sandra_aamodt_why_dieting_doesn_t_usually_work

- *Teach Every Child About Food*—A TED Talk by Jamie Oliver

  http://www.ted.com/talks/jamie_oliver

- The killer American diet that's sweeping the planet by Dean Ornish

  http://www.ted.com/talks/dean_ornish_on_the_world_s_killer_diet

Exercise and fitness programs

A wealth of free exercise videos are available online, with every discipline offered, from yoga to weight lifting.

- Fitness Blender

  www.firnessblender.com

  Hundreds of full-length workout videos including weight training for fat loss, cardio, flexibility stretches and targeted workouts.

- Do Yoga With Me

  www.doyogawithme.com

  Beginner, intermediate and advanced yoga workouts.

- 30 Days of Yoga with Adriene

  https://www.youtube.com/watch?v=oBu-pQG6sTY

  A series from her selection of over 200 yoga videos on YouTube.

USEFUL AND INFORMATIVE WEBSITES

It's a good idea to be familiar with useful websites to find up-to-date information about nutrition and health. Many websites are interactive: you can enter your personal information (height, weight, age) and receive advice about your nutritional requirements. Be careful that your sources are trustworthy, as there is a lot of misinformation out there.

Here are my recommendations for websites from universities, US government agencies and private foundations. You will find a wealth of information at your fingertips.

Nutrition information, portions and fitness trackers

These websites will give you specific nutritional information about food and your suggested daily allowances.

- USDA Food Composition Databases

  https://ndb.nal.usda.govBy the US Department of Agriculture

  A very comprehensive database of nutrition labels from branded foods.

- Choose My Plate

  www.ChooseMyPlate.gov

  By the US Department of Agriculture.

  A wide range of information from dietary guidelines with suggested portions to recipes. You'll also find interactive online tools including: daily checklists, supertracker for diet and exercise, and BMI calculator.

- The Nutrition Source

  www.hsph.harvard.edu

  By the Harvard T.H. Chan School of Public Health

  A full spectrum of useful information about nutrition with recommendations.

  Free monthly newsletter.

- My Fitness Pal

  www.myfitnesspal.com

  by UnderArmour Connected Fitness

  One of the most popular websites and apps available for counting calories and tracking your food and exercise, this is also available as an app. Signup is required but it's free.

- US Department of Agriculture National Agricultural Library

  https://fnic.nal.usda.gov

  This extensive website has a useful A-Z index of topics which makes finding information fast and easy. It also has lists of resources from lifecycle nutrition and dietary guidance to food safety.

General health information and healthy living

These websites cover general health information, healthy living or focus on specific concerns. Some have free newsletters which are well-worth receiving.

- Harvard Health Publications

  www.health.harvard.edu

  By Harvard Medical School

  From information about specific diseases to healthy lifestyles, this informative website offers trusted advice.

  Free newsletter.

- American Heart Association

  www.heart.org

  Extensive information about heart disease, stroke and diabetes.

  Free newsletter.

- National Institutes of Health

  www.nih.gov/health-information

  By the US Department of Health & Human Services

  This website is a portal to multiple institutes working on health issues. I especially recommend their pages on weight loss and nutrition myths.

  Telephone advice at the Health Information Center: 800-860-8747

- WebMD

  www.webmd.com

  A very popular, comprehensive website that is easy to use, and offers clear descriptions and practical answers to your health questions. They also offer many online tools for food and fitness planning.

  Free newsletter.

- The Centers for Disease Control & Prevention (CDC)

  www.cdc.gov

  This is the leading national public health institute of the United States.

  In addition to extensive, up-to-date information about diseases and conditions, the CDC also maintains a large section on healthy living which includes US statistics, interactive databases and recommendations about weight and healthy food environments. Strategies for improving the health of communities are also offered.

Sleep and sleep disorders

Because sleep—or lack of it—is so important and influences our hormones and willpower, I recommend these websites.

- National Sleep Foundation

  https://sleepfoundation.org

This is an easy-to-navigate website that covers sleep disorders, travel and sleep recommendations. Video library for easy learning.

- The Stanford Center for Sleep Sciences and Medicine

  sleep.stanford.edu

  The website from the Stanford University School of Medicine, offers reports on their research on sleep and sleep disorders such as apnea, insomnia and nighttime sleep behaviors. Appointments at the sleep clinic are available.

Weight loss and eating disorders

These websites focus on the consequences, both positive and negative, of weight loss.

- The National Weight Control Registry

  www.nwcronline.com

  Founded by two doctors in 1994, this organization has tracked over 10,000 people who have lost at least 30 pounds and kept it off for a year. Their research findings of successful practices are available online, along with inspiring success stories. You can join the registry if you are over 18 and fit their weight loss criterion.

- National Eating Disorders Association

  www.nationaleatingdisorders.org

  Not all focus on losing weight is healthy. This websites offers general information about eating disorders and a hot line to offer help and support for individuals and families. 800-931-2237

Food policy and our national food supply

The American food supply touches everyone and keeping our food safe and healthy is of vital importance. Here are my recommendations for websites and blogs from trusted researchers, institutions and journalists.

- Food Politics

  www.foodpolitics.com

By Marion Nestle, Palette Goddard Professor in the Department of Nutrition, Food Studies and Public Health at New York University. A daily blog which covers industry practices and most recent nutrition research. Subscribe for free.

- US Food and Drug Administration

www.FDA.gov

The government agency that sets rules for nutrition fact labels. This huge website food-borne illness and how to start a food business.

- Cooking for a healthy lifestyle

The web is full of captivating cooking websites. These focus on healthy meals that feature vegetables, lean meats, low sugar recipes.

- Inspiralized

www.inspiralized.com

Recipes for turning vegetables into healthy, delicious meals. You will need a kitchen tool to spiralize fibrous vegetables.

- Vegetarian cooking

www.pinterest.com/explore/vegetarian-cooking

Thousands of vegetarian recipes from around the world

On www.youtube.com search for these terms:

Meal prep, low-fat cooking, low-carb cooking, sugar-free recipes

Go to

www.WeightControlThatWorks.com

for more valuable information about
how to lose weight and keep it off.

ABOUT THE AUTHOR

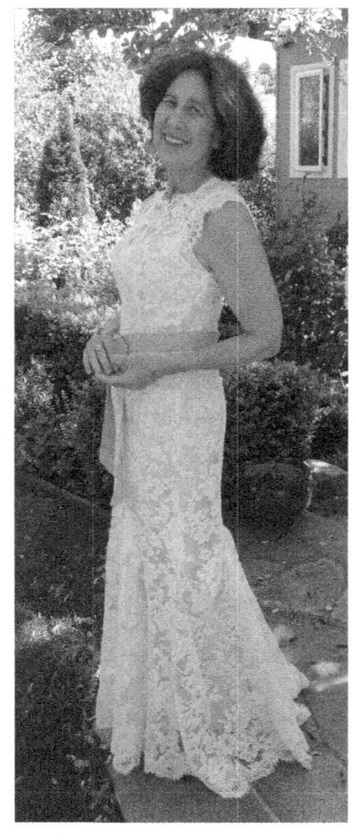

Christie Jordan writes for people who wish to reinvent their lives. She's an entrepreneur and product designer with over 30 years of experience as the CEO of an international design and manufacturing company, inventing and launching products for Fortune 500 companies. She studied at the University of California, Berkeley, and the Harvard Business School. Throughout her adult life, Christie struggled with her weight, gaining and losing through yo-yo diets, until she finally figured out how to lose 85 pounds and keep them off permanently. She lives with her family in the San Francisco Bay Area.

Contact Christie at
www.HopefulWoman.com

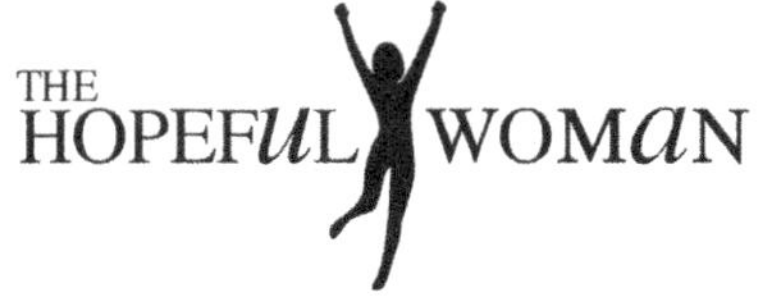

INDEX

Made in the USA
Monee, IL
07 July 2026

56551154R00174